VITAMINS AND MINERALS

Questions
you
have
... Answers
you
need

Other Books From The People's Medical Society

Take This Book to the Hospital With You

How to Evaluate and Select a Nursing Home

Medicine on Trial

Medicare Made Easy

Your Medical Rights

Getting the Most for Your Medical Dollar

Take This Book to the Gynecologist With You

Take This Book to the Obstetrician With You

Healthy Body Book: Test Yourself for Maximum Health

Blood Pressure: Questions You Have . . . Answers You Need

Your Heart: Questions You Have . . . Answers You Need

The Consumer's Guide to Medical Lingo

150 Ways to Be a Savvy Medical Consumer

Take This Book to the Pediatrician With You

100 Ways to Live to 100

Dial 800 for Health

Your Complete Medical Record

Arthritis: Questions You Have . . . Answers You Need

Diabetes: Questions You Have . . . Answers You Need

Prostate: Questions You Have . . . Answers You Need

Good Operations—Bad Operations

VITAMINS AND MINERALS

Questions you have ...Answers you need

By Ellen Moyer

≡People's Medical Society.

Allentown, Pennsylvania

The People's Medical Society is a nonprofit consumer health organization dedicated to the principles of better, more responsive and less expensive medical care. Organized in 1983, the People's Medical Society puts previously unavailable medical information into the hands of consumers so that they can make informed decisions about their own health care.

Membership in the People's Medical Society is $20 a year and includes a subscription to the *People's Medical Society Newsletter.* For information, write to the People's Medical Society, 462 Walnut Street, Allentown, PA 18102, or call 610-770-1670.

This and other People's Medical Society publications are available for quantity purchase at discount. Contact the People's Medical Society for details.

© 1993 by the People's Medical Society
Printed in the United States of America

Library of Congress Cataloging-in-Publication Data
Moyer, Ellen.
    Vitamins and minerals : questions you have, answers you need / by Ellen Moyer.
        p. cm.
    Includes bibliographical references and index.
    ISBN 1-882606-05-1
    1. Vitamins in human nutrition—Miscellanea.   2. Minerals in human nutrition—Miscellanea.   3. Health—Miscellanea.   I. Title.
RA784.M68   1993
613.2'8—dc20   93-30754
                                                                              CIP

            6 7 8 9 0
First printing, September 1993

CONTENTS

INTRODUCTION

It is hard to believe that the topic of vitamins and minerals would be controversial. But the only thing "experts" seem to agree on when discussing the subject is that humans have a daily need for certain vitamins and minerals. After that the arguments begin. How much of a particular nutrient does a person need? Do some people need more than others do? Should our sources of vitamins and minerals be foods alone? Should we augment our diets by taking vitamins and minerals in pill, liquid or other form? What about megadoses of vitamins for certain conditions? Can such megadoses prevent diseases or lessen their impact?

The controversies surrounding vitamins and minerals spread even to the federal government. Battles are ongoing over the process the government uses to determine its guidelines for daily minimum requirements. There have been major disputes about whether vitamins should be classified as a food (the current status) or drug (thus requiring control and physician prescription).

All this leaves most consumers confused. Turn on Oprah Winfrey one day and listen to an advocate claiming that a megadose of one nutrient cured a child of a fatal disease. Turn on Phil Donahue the next day and listen to someone suggesting that a megadose of the same product does not cure anything but instead is toxic.

In *Vitamins and Minerals: Questions You Have . . . Answers You Need,* all the questions about vitamins and minerals most consumers have are answered. We have attempted to provide you with the widest range of unbiased information possible to help you better understand the role and use of vitamins and minerals in your daily diet and life.

Vitamins and Minerals: Questions You Have . . . Answers You Need is another book in a long series of books from the People's Medical Society designed to inform and empower the health-care consumer. The information in this book comes directly from the foremost sources in health and medical literature. It is our goal to help you better understand the role of vitamins and minerals in your daily life, and to assist you in meeting your nutritional needs.

Veteran health writer Ellen Moyer has done extensive research to bring you the latest and most updated information about the topics covered in this book. Her vision has been to bring clarity to what is often a chaotic subject. There is no doubt she has realized that goal.

Charles B. Inlander
President
People's Medical Society

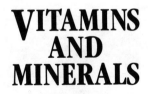

VITAMINS AND MINERALS

Questions
you
have
... Answers
you
need

Terms printed in boldface can be found in the glossary, beginning on page 201. Only the first mention of the word in the text will be boldfaced.

We have tried to use male and female pronouns in an egalitarian manner throughout the book. Any imbalance in usage has been in the interest of readability.

1 NUTRITION AND THE ROLES OF VITAMINS AND MINERALS

Q: It seems that not so long ago the only people interested in nutrition were home-economics teachers and, maybe, Mom. Now the topic is making the covers of national news magazines and the front page of the *New York Times.* Why is nutrition such a hot topic these days? And what do **vitamins** and **minerals** have to do with it?

A: Critics say that our current fascination with nutrition is merely a media-fed craze concocted by the vitamin-supplement industry to strike a chord with aging baby boomers, but that's nowhere near the truth.

Nutrition is a hot topic right now for good reason. Within the last 10 years or so, researchers have been conducting impressive new nutrition studies in the United States. This research goes light-years beyond our previous understanding of the role nutrition plays in health.

Q: Who's doing such research?

A: Prestigious research centers, such as the National Cancer Institute, the U.S. Department of Agriculture Human Nutrition Research Centers and the American Institute for Cancer Research, as well as dozens of well-known universities, such as Harvard, Tufts, the University of Alabama, the University of Texas and campuses of the University of California at Berkeley, San Diego and San Francisco. Plus, it has attracted scientists from around the world.

Q: What is all this research looking at?

A: Researchers have been exploring many different aspects of nutrition: the benefits and hazards of different kinds of fats, such as saturated fats, fish oils and hydrogenated fats (the hardened vegetable oils found in margarine, for example); the role of different types of fibers in reducing cholesterol and cutting the risks of colon and breast cancers; and the reasons behind the fact that people who eat large quantities of fruits and vegetables seem to have reduced risk for many kinds of disease.

Q: Okay, but what do vitamins and minerals have to do with this?

A: As researchers isolate food components that seem to protect against, say, heart disease and cancer, they are discovering that vitamins and minerals play an important role in providing that protection—a role beyond what was previously thought. Vitamins and minerals are certainly not the only components of food that offer health benefits, but they are proving to be an important part.

Q: What kinds of benefits are you talking about?

A: Scientists who thought that the major benefits of **nutrients** were to prevent **deficiency-related diseases**, such as **rickets**, **beriberi** and **scurvy**, are learning that vitamins and minerals play far more funda-mental and long-term roles in the body than anybody had previously suspected.

Specifically, they are gathering evidence that vitamins and minerals influence the health of nearly every organ and may slow or even reverse many diseases previously thought an inevitable part of aging, such as cancer, heart disease, **osteo-porosis**, impaired immunity, nerve degeneration and other chronic health problems.

Q: Can you give me some examples of this evidence you're talking about?

A: Throughout this book, as we discuss specific nutrients, we present such evidence, but here are some broad examples. High intakes of **vitamins C** and **E**, and **beta-carotene** (the orange pigment found in carrots and other vegetables and fruits) are linked with reduced deaths from cancer and heart disease. High intakes of **potassium**, **magnesium** and **calcium** are all associated with lower blood pressure. High intake of **folic acid** decreases a woman's chances of having a baby with serious birth defects and also reduces her risk of developing cervical abnormalities that can lead to cancer.

Q: What do you mean by high intake?

A: In general, high intake means intake that is above average relative to the general population. If most of the people in a group are getting about 70 milligrams of vitamin C a day, for instance, people getting more than that amount would be considered a high-intake group.

Q: And what about low intake?

A: In general, it means below-average intake of a particular nutrient relative to the general population. You see, in population studies, scientists usually divide the people they are studying into low-, medium-, high- and very-high nutrient-intake groups. The high- and very-high intake groups are then compared with the low-intake group for differences in disease risk. From such studies, scientists come up with amounts of nutrients that seem to offer protective benefits.

Q: Can you tell me more about this research?

A: Research has been worldwide and has included hundreds of population studies that examine and compare the eating habits and patterns of illness among large numbers of people. These studies are designed to reveal associations between certain eating habits, nutrient intakes and disease risks. For instance, dozens of studies now show that people who eat a lot of fruits and vegetables suffer fewer of certain types of cancer than people whose intake of fruits and vegetables is low.

Q: How many servings a day of fruits and vegetables do these studies consider "a lot"?

A: In most of these studies, four or more servings a day of fruits or vegetables qualifies as "a lot."

Q: And how many servings a day of fruits or vegetables is considered a low intake?

A: One or no servings a day is considered low intake.

Q: What's a serving?

A: This may vary from study to study, but, in general, a serving is one medium fruit, 6 ounces of 100 percent fruit or vegetable juice, ½ cup cooked or raw vegetables or fruit, one cup of raw leafy vegetables or ¼ cup dried fruit.

Q: How do researchers test such findings?

A: In addition to years of animal research, researchers have recently moved into what are called "human clinical intervention trials." Some of these studies add a nutrient to the diets of people at risk for a certain disorder to see if it helps prevent development of the disorder. Others add a nutrient to the diets of generally healthy people to see if it improves certain aspects of their health, such as immune function.

Q: Any noteworthy results yet from these human clinical intervention trials?

A: Researchers at several cancer centers have found that the same **synthetic** vitamin A-like substance used to treat severe acne, **isotretinoin** (brand name Accutane) helps to prevent a recurrence of leukoplakia, a precancerous condition of the mouth that often afflicts smokers.

And as we touched upon earlier, researchers now know that supplemental folic acid, a B vitamin, reduces a woman's risk of having a baby with **neural-tube defects**, serious birth defects that result in spinal-cord and brain abnormalities.

Q: Anything else?

A: Researchers have found that vitamin B6 supplements can boost immunity in older people, who apparently may need more than currently recommended amounts of this nutrient to maintain adequate body stores.

Many other studies, now ongoing, should produce results in several more years. One particular study, by researchers at the University of Texas Health Sciences Center, in Tyler, Texas, is testing whether high doses of supplemental beta-carotene help prevent lung cancer in smokers who have been exposed to asbestos.

Another, by researchers in the United States and China, is looking to see if supplementing people's diets with **selenium**, a trace mineral, reduces the high rates of cancer in people living in certain areas of China where soil levels of selenium are low. And several researchers are investigating whether giving people at risk for colon cancer up to five grams a day of calcium reduces their risk of developing potentially pre-malignant intestinal polyps.

Q: What happens once the results of these studies are in?

A: The results can help guide researchers in further studies and provide information that helps people make decisions regarding diet and supplementation. But more such studies are probably needed to clarify the roles of vitamins and minerals in disease prevention.

"We know that years of eating the right kind of diet seems to protect people from certain types of cancer and other diseases, but we still don't know whether we can do anything to overcome a lifetime of risks with just a short period of supplementation, even at fairly high levels," says Jerry McLarty, Ph.D., who is directing the University of Texas lung-cancer study.

"Every researcher in this area has had to deal with a lot of unknowns: how much of a nutrient to give, how long to give it, and the like. That's what some of these studies are trying to figure out."

VITAMINS

Q: Sounds interesting, but let's back up. I know very little about nutrition and even less about vitamins and minerals. So let's start at the beginning. What exactly are vitamins?

A: Vitamins are nutrients—food components obtained from our diets—that have been found to be essential in small quantities for human life. This means that if even one vitamin is missing from your diet, your body does not function normally.

Vitamins are a group of chemically unrelated organic substances. Organic substances are compounds containing the chemical element carbon and they come only from living materials—plants or animals, or from substances that were once living materials, such as petroleum oil or coal.

Q: What do vitamins do?

A: Vitamins perform countless different functions in the body, and individual vitamins have special functions. As a group, however, most of them share in certain functions, such as the promotion of growth, the promotion of the ability to produce healthy offspring and the maintenance of health. They must be present for the body to be able to utilize other essential nutrients, such as minerals, **fatty acids**, **amino acids** and energy sources (for example, **carbohydrates** and **sugar**). Vitamins are also important to a normal appetite and digestive tract, to mental alertness, to health of tissues and to resistance to bacterial infections.

Q: How do vitamins do all those things?

A: Our bodies use vitamins to make substances called **coenzymes**. Coenzymes are vital participants in many of the ongoing chemical reactions in our bodies that, in fact, are the very essence of life. These chemical reactions provide our body's cells with energy from food—a process called **metabolism**. These chemical reactions allow cells to grow and divide, promoting growth in children and tissue repair in adults. They also allow our bodies to quickly build up a supply of infection-fighting immune cells when necessary.

If you lack even one vitamin, you may fail to thrive as a child or be smaller than normal and may fail to develop sexually. As an adult, if you lack a vitamin, you eventually develop a deficiency-related disease, such as scurvy (from lack of vitamin C) or rickets (from lack of vitamin D), and you are more vulnerable to infection. Exactly what health problem you develop depends on which vitamin you are lacking.

Q: I know from reading my kitty's "chow" bag that cats need vitamins, too. But do animals need the same vitamins that humans need?

A: All animals need some vitamins, but not every vitamin that has been discovered to be essential for humans is also needed by every animal. There are, however, more similarities than differences. Here's one interesting difference: Unlike humans, most animals can make vitamin C in their bodies, so they do not need to get this vitamin from food. Guinea pigs are the exception, which is why they were used as animal models for studies where humans could not be used (for proving the ability of vitamin C to prevent scurvy).

Humans, however, can make **vitamin D** in their bodies. And some of the vitamin needs of animals and humans can be supplied from **microorganisms** living in the digestive tract.

Q: What? We have *things* living in our bodies that make vitamins for us?

A: Yes. But while that fact may be startling it's not as bad as you think. Indeed, this is a healthy state of affairs. All humans have bacteria, also called **microflora** or microorganisms, living in their intestines, and these bacteria can **synthesize**, or produce, certain amounts of vitamins **K**, **B**$_{12}$ and **biotin**, which are absorbed through the intestines. In most cases, however, we also rely on food sources of these vitamins to stay healthy.

Q: I know this may sound silly, but what about other living things, such as plants? Do they need vitamins, too?

A: Most plants do not require vitamins. Some of what scientists call "lower plant forms"—bacteria and yeast—do need an outside source for some vitamins. Minerals are an entirely different story, and we'll get to them shortly.

Q: What does the word vitamin mean?

A: The word *vitamine* was coined in 1912 by Polish biochemist Casimir Funk, who first proposed the theory that disease might be caused by a lack of something in the diet and cured by adding it back. Believe it or not, this line of thinking was considered novel at that time, since many in the medical community were so smitten by Joseph Lister's new "germ theory" of disease that they couldn't conceive of a disease being caused by a lack of something in the diet.

Funk thought this missing substance was necessary for life (*vita*) and contained nitrogen (*amine*). Subsequent work showed that although there were many "vitamines," few contained nitrogen. So the "e" was dropped, giving us vitamin.

Q: How many vitamins are there?

A: There are 13 known vitamins. Four are fat-soluble—A, D, E and K; and nine are water-soluble—the B vitamins and vitamin C. The B vitamins essential for human health are B_1, or **thiamin**; B_2, or **riboflavin**; **niacin**; B_6; B_{12}, or **cobalamin**; folic acid; **pantothenic acid**, and biotin.

Q: Why the distinction between fat- and water-soluble vitamins? Is it important only to researchers?

A: It's important to researchers because it helps them identify the functions of these vitamins. As for the rest of us, we should know that fat-soluble vitamins need a bit of fat in the diet to be absorbed and that, if for some reason we're taking supplements of these vitamins, it is best to take them with a meal that contains some fat. We should also know that fat-soluble vitamins tend to stay in the body longer than most water-soluble vitamins, so some of the fat-soluble vitamins can build up to unhealthy levels more easily than most water-soluble vitamins can. These toxic levels are likely to be reached only by taking supplements or by eating foods exceptionally rich in a particular nutrient.

Q: Are those all the vitamins there are?

A: There are other substances that are occasionally considered to be essential vitamins. Their vitamin status, however, has not been established. These substances include **choline, inositol, bioflavonoids, para-aminobenzoic acid (PABA)** and a few others.

Q: What does that mean—"their vitamin status has not been established"?

A: These are nutrients that may be vitamins for certain species, that humans require under certain conditions not yet understood, or that have functions not yet understood. We talk more about these so-called **quasi-vitamins** a little later.

Q: Beta-carotene is getting a lot of public attention these days, yet you didn't list it as one of the one of the 13 known vitamins. Is it one of the quasi-vitamins?

A: No. Beta-carotene is a **precursor** to **vitamin A**. In other words, it's a substance from which vitamin A can be made. We discuss its role in more detail in the section on vitamin A in Chapter 8.

Q: You said that vitamins are involved in energy metabolism. Do they provide energy?

A: Vitamins don't provide energy, but some are fundamental participants in the energy-producing reactions of our bodies—the reactions that help our cells burn sugar or fat to make energy. Vitamins themselves, however, are insignificant sources of biological energy.

Q: Before we go on, what exactly is the process of metabolism?

A: Metabolism usually refers to a complex chemical process that involves the breakdown and release of energy from food. The metabolic process allows our bodies to convert food calories (carbohydrates, sugar and fat) into usable energy.

In a greater sense, metabolism also includes all the many physical and chemical processes by which living, organized substances, including the cells in our bodies, are built up and maintained.

Q: So what happens if we don't have enough of a vitamin for metabolism?

A: If a vitamin is in short supply, metabolism may not be completed. You may suffer from fatigue as a result of the inability to supply your body with energy; and you may develop health problems, as improperly metabolized fats, proteins, carbohydrates and sugars build up in your cells or blood.

Q: How do we get vitamins?

A: Part of the definition of a vitamin is that it must be obtained, at least in part, from outside the body, since we cannot make vitamins in our bodies in adequate amounts. We obtain vitamins from the foods we eat—including vitamin-enriched foods—and from vitamin supplements.

Q: Do all foods contain vitamins?

A: Just about every food we eat contains at least some vitamins, but some are much better sources than others.

Some foods considered as traditional health foods—liver, blackstrap molasses, brown rice, wheat germ, eggs, **brewer's yeast** and kale, for instance—contain an impressive array of vitamins and minerals.

And other foods provide large amounts of one particular vitamin. Citrus fruits and red peppers are loaded with vitamin C, for example; wheat-germ oil is a good source of vitamin E; and parsley is packed with vitamin K.

Q: Are there any foods that don't contain vitamins?

A: Although they provide more than enough calories, certain foods, such as sugar, animal fat (lard), soda and alcohol, are devoid of vitamins. They are what **nutritionists** and **dietitians** call "empty calories." In fact, they're worse than that, since these foods require vitamins and minerals to be metabolized. So they use up important nutrients in our bodies without replacing them. Eating a lot of sugar or fat or having more than a drink or two of alcohol a day increases your vitamin needs, which puts you at increased risk for developing vitamin deficiencies.

Q: It sounds like we'd all be better off eating brown rice and seaweed if we want to get vitamins. Is that the case?

A: Your diet need not be that severe to get the nutrients you need. But the general rule is that the less processed a food is, the more nutrients it retains. That goes for vitamins and minerals. **Enriched** processed foods do replace some of the vitamins and minerals lost during processing, and **fortified** foods may contain nutrients they never had in the first place. But we're getting ahead of ourselves. We discuss enriched and fortified foods in more detail later.

Q: You also said we can get vitamins as supplements. Are the vitamins we get from pills the same as the vitamins found in foods?

A: For the most part, they are exactly the same. More on vitamin and mineral supplements later.

MINERALS

Q: Okay, now I know something about vitamins. What are minerals?

A: Minerals, such as calcium, magnesium and **iron**, are nonorganic compounds. That means that, unlike vitamins, mineral molecules do not contain carbon and do not originate from living organisms.

Q: Then how do we get minerals—by eating rocks?

A: Indirectly. People obtain minerals from the plant or animal foods they eat, and from water, which may contain dissolved minerals. Supplementation is another way to get minerals.

Q: You've already mentioned several minerals. Which ones do we need?

A: There are 15 that are currently considered essential for humans: calcium, magnesium, **phosphorus**, **sodium**, potassium, **sulfur, chlorine**, iron, **iodine, copper, manganese, zinc, molybdenum**, selenium and **chromium**.

Q: How does an inorganic compound, such as a mineral, get into plants, which are organic?

A: Plants obtain minerals from the soil in which they are grown. Plants grown in soil deficient in a certain mineral will themselves be low in that mineral. In a certain region of China, for instance, the soil lacks selenium; therefore, people's diets are poor in this essential **trace mineral**. These people also have a high incidence of cardiomyopathy (a disease of the heart muscle) and of cancers of the stomach, esophagus and liver. Studies in China, where selenium supplements were added to the diet, are helping to prove that selenium is essential to human health and to pin down required amounts.

Q: You mentioned the term trace mineral. What is that?

A: Trace minerals are minerals that we need only in traces, or very small amounts. Minerals are often grouped in two categories: those required in our diets in amounts greater than 100 milligrams a day and those required in amounts less than 100 milligrams a day. Those minerals that we require in large amounts (greater than 100 milligrams a day) are referred to simply as minerals. Those we need in small amounts (less than 100 milligrams) are called trace minerals. There are even minerals called **ultra-trace minerals**—those, such as molybdenum, that may be needed in fractions of milligrams.

Q: I've also seen the term **trace element**. Is a trace element the same as a trace mineral?

A: Yes. Both words have the same meaning and are interchangeable.

Q: Are some foods higher in minerals than other foods?

A: Yes. Minerals are present in most foods in varying amounts. Dairy products, for instance, are an excellent source of calcium, as well as some potassium and magnesium. Fruits and vegetables provide potassium, magnesium and sometimes calcium. Meats, poultry and fish contain iron, zinc, copper and other trace minerals, while whole grains contribute magnesium, iron, zinc, copper and other trace minerals.

Even some herbs and spices are highly concentrated sources of trace minerals. The herb thyme, for instance, contains 100 times as much chromium as meat does, and 400 times as much manganese. Black pepper, cloves, ginger and bay leaves are all rich sources of trace minerals. In fact, it's been suggested that their richness in taste is due to their concentration of such minerals.

Q: So what foods *don't* supply minerals?

A: Foods that contain no appreciable amounts of minerals include animal fats, oils, sugar, alcohol and—unless they are enriched—refined grains, such as white flour.

Q: What do minerals do?

A: Even though they might be receiving less public attention these days than vitamins, minerals are as important as vitamins for our bodies to function properly. Like vitamins, dietary minerals participate in many biochemical and physiological processes necessary for good health.

For instance, calcium, the mineral we think of as important for strong bones, also plays a major role in blood-pressure regulation, blood clotting, the maintenance of muscle tone and the normal rhythmical contraction of the heart.

Iron, generally known for its important role in carrying oxygen throughout the body, is also involved in the proper function of the thyroid gland, in the production of **neuro-transmitters** (chemical substances that allow the brain and nerves to function), in the regulation of body temperature, and in metabolism.

And magnesium, a mineral few of us probably know much about, is known to be part of more than 300 biochemical reactions in the body. It plays a vital role in virtually every body function—from bone development to blood-pressure regulation to proper brain function.

Q: Are there other essential minerals besides those you've mentioned?

A: Possibly. Some trace minerals appear to be important for animals. These are fluorine, tin, boron, vanadium, silicon, nickel, arsenic, cadmium and lead. But what role, if any, these elements play in human nutrition has yet to be determined.

"Much is yet to be learned about the role of minerals, especially trace minerals," admits James Penland, Ph.D., a research psychologist at the USDA Human Nutrition Research Center, at Grand Forks, North Dakota. "Particularly for some of the more esoteric trace minerals, like boron, and even for manganese, little is known about how much is found in foods or how much people actually eat or absorb. Trace minerals exist in foods in such small amounts that the equipment and procedures needed to detect them are fairly sophisticated and expensive."

THE ROLE OF RESEARCH

Q: **How have researchers figured out which vitamins and minerals are essential to life?**

A: The very earliest "research," if you will, was the simple observation that people who eat certain types of restricted diets don't seem to do very well. For instance, it was noted as early as 1498 that sailors who subsisted for months on dried biscuits and salted meat often developed bleeding gums, bruises under the skin, rough skin, joint pain, fatigue, tissue degeneration and increased incidence of infection. This was later discovered to be scurvy, a vitamin C-deficiency disease. For many, this disease was fatal.

Centuries went by, however, before it was accepted that citrus fruits and particularly vitamin C actually did prevent scurvy. Not until 1804 did the British Navy make it a regular practice to issue daily rations of limes to all sailors—a measure that gave rise to the term "limey" as a slang expression for a British seaman. And it wasn't until the 1930s that vitamin C was isolated and synthesized—concocted in a laboratory for purposes of experimentation. Still, its scientific name, **ascorbate**, recalls vitamin C's seafaring past. It means "anti-scurvy."

Q: Any other research of note from centuries ago?

A: Definitely. Scurvy wasn't the only nutrition-related condition observed centuries ago. The writings of ancient Greek, Roman and Arab physicians show that animal liver, rich in vitamin A, was known to be effective in both the prevention and cure of night blindness, a condition now known to be caused by vitamin A deficiency. And as early as 2600 B.C., Chinese scholars noted symptoms, such as **peripheral** nerve degeneration, heart enlargement and fluid retention, in Asian populations subsisting on polished rice. Such symptoms are consistent with beriberi, a thiamin-deficiency disease. (Brown rice is a good source of thiamin; unenriched white rice is not.)

Q: Well, so much for observations. What about modern science?

A: Two factors had to be in place before researchers could begin what we think of as modern nutrition science, says Gerald F. Combs Jr., Ph.D., a professor of nutrition at Cornell University, in Ithaca, New York.

First, researchers had to know enough about the elements of a diet to be able to make up a purified diet. Diets of this type were formulated using highly refined ingredients, such as isolated proteins, refined sugar and starches, and refined fats. Such diets allowed researchers to control and repeat experiments.

Second, researchers had to find animal models. The first of these animals was discovered by chance by a keen observer, according to Dr. Combs.

Q: What animal was that?

A: The chicken. And here's how it happened: A researcher, Christine Eijkman, was looking for a germ that caused beriberi. He happened to raise chickens but ran out of brown rice and had to feed them polished white rice until another shipment of brown rice arrived months later. In the meantime, many of the chickens developed symptoms that were suspiciously similar to beriberi. When he found that feeding the chickens their usual course of brown rice reversed their symptoms, he began using the chickens for his studies and eventually proved that something in rice hulls protected against this disease.

Q: **Is this typical of the way early research went about?**

A: To a certain extent. For most vitamins and minerals, the research process involved isolating a substance from foods, feeding animals diets deficient in that substance, seeing if they developed a disease, feeding them the missing substance to see if the disease went away, and, in some instances, giving the same substance to humans who appeared to have the disease. Chemical analysis and synthetic manufacture of a vitamin usually occurred years after the substance was initially isolated and identified.

Q: **Do the letters in vitamin names—A, B, C and so on—have to do with the order in which they were discovered?**

A: Well, they were meant to be, but science is not always as orderly as we would like it to be. Vitamin A was discovered first, but the B vitamins kind of mixed things up. Researchers initially thought there was only one B vitamin. They called it water-soluble B. Later, however, they realized that what they thought was one molecule was several, and so, some of the B vitamins were given letters and numbers.

These days, researchers prefer to drop the number designations and refer to vitamins by their proper names. You might see B6 listed as pyridoxine on a vitamin-bottle label, for instance. The B vitamin group is known as **B complex**.

Vitamin K is so named because its Danish discoverers found that it was necessary for blood clotting—*k*oagulation in Danish.

Q: How do researchers determine what amounts of a vitamin or mineral are necessary for good health?

A: Most research to determine the amount of a nutrient that is necessary for good health has been based on the absence of the physical symptoms associated with deficiency. The amount of a nutrient that prevents deficiency-related symptoms in most people is considered an adequate amount.

More recently, however, researchers have started looking at the amounts of nutrients needed for optimum health—the amounts needed for the most resistance to cancer and infection, the lowest risk of diabetes and heart disease, even the longest possible life. Those amounts are considered optimum levels. Optimum levels have yet to be determined for many nutrients, and researchers and public health officials frequently scrap over what amounts should be officially recommended.

VITAMINS AND MINERALS IN DAILY DIET

Q: Can I get all the vitamins and minerals I need from the foods I eat?

A: It is possible to obtain an adequate amount of every nutrient through food. It's not easy, though, and requires both planning and eating a minimum number of calories from nutrient-rich sources each day.

Optimal amounts of some nutrients, such as vitamin E, however, are impossible to attain through a normal diet. Even if you're eating plenty of vitamin E-rich vegetable oils and nuts, a diet of about 2,500 calories would provide, at most, 40 to 50 international units, or I.U., of vitamin E. Some trace-mineral researchers also contend that ideal amounts of trace minerals, such as chromium, are impossible to obtain through diets containing fewer than 4,000 to 5,000 calories a day.

Q: How much I eat each day makes a big difference in whether I get all the vitamins and minerals I need?

A: It does, along with the foods you select to eat. More often than men, women tend to fall short on vitamins and minerals because they are on calorie-restricted diets. Most nutritionists agree that if you're eating fewer than 1,800 to 2,000 calories a day, you're unlikely to get all the vitamins and minerals you need, even with a carefully planned diet. In fact, you're likely to get less of many vitamins and minerals than you need. That may not hurt you if you're dieting for only a few weeks, but if you stick to such a diet for a few months, you could start experiencing fatigue or other problems related to nutritional deficiencies, experts say. That's one reason many diet programs today recommend more calories and about an hour's worth of exercise a day to burn about 300 calories.

Q: So I need to get a certain quantity of food. But what about quality? What foods should I eat to make sure I get the vitamins and minerals I need?

A: Across the board, nutrition experts stress eating a varied diet, one that contains foods from all the food groups, and within those groups, a creative mix-and-match that broadens your range of selection, from apples to kiwi, kohlrabi to yams.

Q: Food groups? I've heard of the Basic Four Food Groups, but I don't remember what they are. Also, haven't these groups been replaced by something different?

A: The Basic Four Food Groups, dietary guidelines developed by the U.S. Department of Agriculture (USDA) and taught for many years in public schools, divided foods into—no surprise—four groups: milk, meat, vegetables and fruit, and cereals.

Concern that the Basic Four Food Groups put too much weight on high-fat meats and dairy products, coupled with new research showing the health benefits of a high-fiber, grain- and vegetable-based diet, led to the development of new dietary guidelines and to a new teaching tool called the Food Pyramid—also courtesy of the USDA.

Q: What are the new USDA guidelines?

A: The new guidelines break foods into six groups and recommend you eat a certain number of servings from each group each day—except for the fats, oils and sweets groups, which they suggest you use sparingly. These guidelines are represented by the Food Pyramid pictured below.

Food Guide Pyramid
A Guide to Daily Food Choices

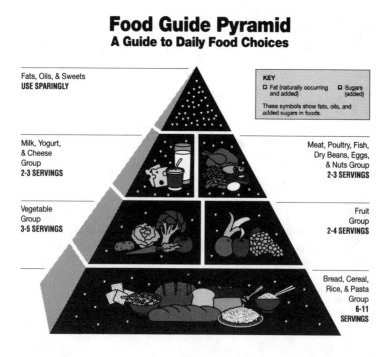

Fats, Oils, & Sweets
USE SPARINGLY

KEY
□ Fat (naturally occurring and added)   □ Sugars (added)
These symbols show fats, oils, and added sugars in foods.

Milk, Yogurt, & Cheese Group
2-3 SERVINGS

Meat, Poultry, Fish, Dry Beans, Eggs, & Nuts Group
2-3 SERVINGS

Vegetable Group
3-5 SERVINGS

Fruit Group
2-4 SERVINGS

Bread, Cereal, Rice, & Pasta Group
6-11 SERVINGS

Q: What is considered a serving size?

A: For milk, yogurt and cheese: 1 cup of milk or yogurt, 1½ ounces of natural cheese or 2 ounces of processed cheese. For meat: 2 to 3 ounces of cooked lean meat, fish or poultry; 1 to 1½ cups cooked dry beans, 2 to 3 eggs, and 4 to 6 tablespoons of peanut butter. For vegetables: 1 cup raw, leafy vegetables, ½ cup other vegetables (cooked or chopped raw) or ¾ cup vegetable juice. For fruit: 1 medium apple, banana or orange; ½ cup chopped, cooked or canned fruit; ¾ cup fruit juice. For bread, cereal, rice and pasta: 1 slice of bread, 1 ounce of ready-to-eat cereal, or ½ cup cooked cereal, rice or pasta.

Q: What about other guidelines? Haven't other government and private agencies also issued guidelines on how to eat?

A: Yes. Several sets of guidelines exist, but they are pretty much the same. In addition to the Food Pyramid recommendations, for instance, the USDA and U.S. Department of Health and Human Services together offer these recommendations:

- Eat a variety of foods.

- Maintain healthy weight.

- Choose a diet low in fat, saturated fat and cholesterol.

- Choose a diet with plenty of vegetables, fruits and grain products.

- Use sugar and salt only in moderation.

- If you drink alcoholic beverages, do so in moderation.

Q: Why does the federal government feel it needs to address how people eat? Don't people in the United States eat pretty well, at least compared with most countries?

A: Americans certainly have the opportunity to eat more food than people in many countries, but that doesn't necessarily mean they are eating well. Eating too much, especially of fats, sugar, salt and calories, has been linked with many of the chronic diseases to which Americans are prone. And because so many tax dollars go toward medical care for these diseases, the U.S. government no doubt feels it is in its best interest to get people to eat better.

Q: How do Americans eat?

A: Poorly, for the most part, according to the latest score-cards on the subject. A recent study from the University of California at Berkeley showed that only 2 percent of Americans are keeping their fat intake below 30 percent of calories and getting at least two-thirds of the recommended amounts for nutrients each day. The survey also showed that only 22 percent of us get at least two-thirds of all the recommended amounts of vitamins and minerals, and that only 14 percent have reached the not very low fat goal of 30 percent or less.

No single age, gender, race or demographic group eats particularly well, according to the California study, but several groups appear to have their own unique dietary vices: alcohol for young men, too few calories and nutrients for young women.

This study also points out that high-fat diets are linked with inadequate vitamin and mineral intake, because fats add a lot of calories to a diet but provide essentially no vitamins or minerals. Only vegetable oils provide some vitamin E. A recent study that looked at vitamin E intake showed that most people got their vitamin E from oil-laden pies and baked goods, although a small percentage of people got large amounts of vitamin E and other vitamins and minerals from fortified breakfast cereals.

Q: So while food is the best way of getting us our vitamins and minerals, it's obvious we don't eat enough of the right foods to ward off deficiency problems. What other ways can we meet our vitamin and mineral needs?

A: One source is through enriched and fortified foods. And that's the subject of our next chapter.

2 ENRICHED AND FORTIFIED FOODS

Q: **You've mentioned several times that vitamins and minerals are sometimes added to foods. What's that all about?**

A: Adding vitamins and minerals to certain foods, either enrichment or fortification, is a common practice in the United States and other countries. Enrichment, you'll recall, involves putting back nutrients lost during processing. Fortification involves beefing up a food with more nutrients than it would have naturally. White rice with added iron and B vitamins is labeled "enriched" because some of the nutrients lost during processing were restored. Orange juice with added calcium, on the other hand, is considered a fortified food because orange juice contains little calcium in its natural state.

Q: **Do you mean that vitamins and minerals are added to foods because people need the nutrients?**

A: In some cases, yes, vitamins and/or minerals are added to selected, widely used foods to ensure that the population gets enough of the nutrient.

For instance, in the United States, iodine has been added to salt since 1924, and this addition has just about wiped out what used to be a fairly common problem in some states: **goiter**, an enlargement of the thyroid gland as a result of iodine deficiency. Slightly less than one-half teaspoon of iodized salt provides enough iodine to prevent goiter. Not all salt contains iodine, however. Manufacturers are required by law to offer both iodized and noniodized versions, and kosher salt is not iodized.

Milk was selected in 1929 to be the carrier for vitamin D, and in just a few years this fortification program had cut the incidence of rickets, a disease of bone malformation, in small children from 16 percent down to 7 percent. Fortified milk has 400 I.U. of vitamin D per quart, the recommended amount.

Vitamin A was added to skim and low-fat milk in the 1940s when this vitamin was found to improve immune response in children and women. Vitamin A is not added to whole milk, which naturally contains some vitamin A. A quart of whole milk provides about one-third of the vitamin A you need each day.

In some communities, municipal water is the carrier of fluoride, a mineral that helps strengthen children's teeth.

Some foods that are considered "substitutes" for other foods are often fortified with the nutrients in those foods. Substitute foods, such as noncitrus fruit drinks (apple juice and fruit punch, for example), may be fortified with vitamin C. Infant formulas and liquid nutritional formulas intended for medical use are required by law to contain certain essential nutrients. Infant formulas, for instance, are formulated to match breast milk in nutrient content.

Q: What about flour? The brands I buy always say enriched on their packages.

A: Compulsory enrichment of bread and flour, introduced in 1942, was replaced after World War II by a voluntary program under state jurisdiction. Currently, most white bread and white flour sold in the United States is enriched with three B complex vitamins—thiamin, riboflavin and niacin—and with iron. White rice is also enriched with these nutrients, and in some states these nutrients are also added to corn meal, corn grits, farina, macaroni and noodles. Whole-wheat flour is not enriched because it naturally contains these nutrients, as well as others.

Q: What about foods that advertisements imply contain every vitamin and mineral under the sun and then some?

A: Some manufacturers add vitamins and minerals to foods as a marketing strategy. A cold cereal, such as Product 19, or a sports bar, such as a PowerBar, boasts an array of vitamins and minerals. There are no regulations regarding such fortification of foods, but "there is usually some sort of rational approach," says Paul Lachance, Ph.D., chairman of the department of food science at Rutgers University, in New Brunswick, New Jersey. "Very few of these foods exceed 100 percent of the RDA. And you can't add something without revealing it on the label."

RDA, or **Recommended Dietary Allowance**, is an amount accepted as adequate. We have more to say about RDAs later.

Q: Are enriched or fortified foods an expensive way to get nutrients?

A: No. They are an inexpensive way to get adequate amounts of certain nutrients, especially for "target populations" (usually women and children), Dr. Lachance says. "Food enrichment is one of the most cost-efficient public-health interventions available," he says. "It's cheaper than taking vitamins as pills." Because of the tonnage involved, it costs only a fraction of a penny to fortify an entire serving of a food with 100 percent of the recommended amount of a nutrient.

Q: Are enriched foods good sources of vitamins and minerals?

A: They are certainly important sources for some nutrients. Most people get about 40 percent of the recommended amount of thiamin from enriched foods, along with about 25 percent of iron, 20 percent of niacin, 15 percent of riboflavin, and 10 percent of vitamins A and C.

"If it weren't for these foods, we would probably still be seeing outright deficiency diseases like **pellagra**, a niacin-deficiency disease, because even with fortification some people are getting only about 10 to 20 percent of the recommended intake from the nutrients that are added to enriched foods," Dr. Lachance says. And people who eat fortified cereals frequently consume enough of a nutrient, such as vitamin E, to move them into a high-intake category associated with reduced risk of disease.

Q: **Any problems with food enrichment?**

A: Even though some nutrients are added back to processed foods, many are not. Take wheat and rice, for example. The white, milled versions of these grains contain anywhere from 20 to 50 percent less of vitamin E, folic acid, pantothenic acid, vitamin B_6, calcium, magnesium, selenium, zinc and other trace minerals than the brown versions.

Q: **Does this mean I shouldn't rely on enriched or fortified foods to meet my nutritional requirements?**

A: You probably are relying on enriched foods to meet some nutritional requirements, whether you are aware of it or not, Dr. Lachance says, unless you are on a strict diet that contains no processed foods.

But you need to keep in mind that enriched foods are lacking certain nutrients you also need. Eating a varied diet that includes, but is not limited to, enriched foods is one way to get the nutrients you need.

Q: But what if I eat a cereal that includes all the vitamins and minerals I need? Won't that be enough?

A: If you rely on a certain fortified food—such as cereal fortified with all the essential vitamins and minerals—to meet your nutritional requirements, you run into the same problem we discuss in the vitamin and mineral supplementation section: There are components in food necessary for good health that are not found in such cereals—fiber, protein, fatty acids and such. Experts recommend that you consider such a food an addition to, not a substitute for, a healthy diet.

Q: Well, you've covered getting vitamins from food, including enriched and fortified foods. What about taking vitamin and mineral supplements?

A: Supplementation is a viable way to get needed vitamins and minerals. Let's look at it in detail.

3 VITAMIN AND MINERAL SUPPLEMENTS

Q: Who takes supplements?

A: About half the people in the United States take nutritional supplements "regularly" or "occasionally," in the words of a national survey by the U.S. Department of Agriculture. The typical user is a woman with at least a high-school education, a higher-than-average income and a better-than-average diet. And she lives in a western state.

Several studies also show supplements are popular among health professionals, including dietitians (who often tell their clients they can get all the nutrients they need from a balanced diet). In one study, 60 percent of dietitians who responded to a mail survey admitted they regularly took supplements, usually multivitamin and mineral products, vitamin C and iron. Some studies also show that supplement use among doctors and medical students is not infrequent. One showed that 14 percent of faculty members at Harvard Medical School usually supplemented their diets. And among medical students at the University of Maryland School of Medicine, more than 60 percent said they took dietary supplements.

Q: Why do people take vitamins?

A: According to one review of studies, it's either because they are uncertain about the nutritional adequacy of their diets, they desire better health than they perceive to be obtainable from medical consultation, or they have decided to treat themselves for an illness.

Frequently given reasons for taking supplements include: "to prevent colds and other illnesses"; "to give me energy"; and "to make up for what is not in food." At least two studies indicate that vitamin users tend to have a low opinion of the quality of today's foods.

Q: Do supplement users report a benefit?

A: Very few studies ask vitamin users whether or not they find supplements helpful. In one that did, 59 percent of people taking vitamins reported they were of "some benefit" to their health and another 34 percent found them to be of "great benefit."

Q: What kinds of vitamins are people taking?

A: According to information from the Council for Responsible Nutrition, a vitamin manufacturers' trade group, sales break down this way:

Multivitamin and mineral supplements	42.0%
Vitamin C	12.2%
Vitamin E	9.6%
B complex	9.1%
Calcium	7.7%
Iron	6.8%
Other vitamins	7.0%
Other minerals	5.6%

And by the way, sales of nutritional supplements have climbed steadily over the years, from $500 million in 1972 to $3.3 billion in 1990.

Q: Health professionals seem concerned that people may harm themselves by overdosing on vitamins and minerals. Does that actually happen much?

A: Not according to information compiled by the Food and Drug Administration (FDA). In 1986 that government agency asked doctors to report any adverse side effects they noted in their patients who took vitamin and mineral supplements. After three years, the agency issued its findings: Only 11 adverse reactions had been reported, and most were minor side effects, such as constipation. In comparison, in that same period of time, the agency received 4,000 reports of adverse reactions from the artificial sweetener aspartame.

Of course, bear in mind that these findings may also mean that doctors are not able to spot and identify such side effects.

Q: How are these rare toxic reactions likely to occur?

A: They seem to fall into one of three categories, says Patricia Hausman, R.D., author of *The Right Dose.* "In about half the cases, toxic reactions are the result of a doctor recommending a large dose of a vitamin or mineral to treat some disease condition, such as large doses of zinc to treat acne," she says. Others occur when too much of a nutrient is added to a food during processing—too much vitamin D in milk, for instance. "Also, some people just do dumb things. But they are few in number," she says. Most adverse effects get better when the high dose of the nutrient is stopped.

One FDA study shows that many vitamin users take most nutrients in amounts that seldom exceeded one to two times the RDA, an amount most experts consider safe. Those taking larger amounts than this are likely to be taking vitamins C and E, which most experts agree are both quite safe, even in large amounts. Some people, however, take up to several hundred times the RDA of several of the B complex vitamins. Those amounts should be taken only with medical supervision, according to experts.

Q: Why do nutritionists stress that vitamin supplements can't make up for a bad diet? I thought that's what they are meant to do.

A: Vitamin and mineral supplements can make up for some nutritional shortcomings, but they can't overcome a lifetime of dietary indiscretions, such as too much fat or salt or too many calories, explains Jacqueline Charnley, R.D., of the USDA Human Nutrition Research Center on Aging, at Tufts University, in Boston.

"There are unknown components of food necessary for good health that just aren't found in a vitamin pill," she says. "And there may be interactions between particular nutrients that depend on food sources. Certainly, too, you need to eat foods to get protein, carbohydrates, fiber, essential fatty acids and some trace minerals that aren't usually found in vitamin pills."

Q: If I decide to take vitamin supplements, how do I figure out what kind to buy? There are so many to choose from, and almost nothing on product labels that would help me make a wise choice.

A: Shopping for supplements can be difficult, no doubt about that. Hundreds of different formulations exist for multivitamin and mineral supplements, and even single-nutrient supplements, such as vitamins C or E, come in a variety of dosages and types. And in health-food stores especially, vitamins and minerals may be mixed with herbs and other nonvitamin ingredients, which can make the selection even more bewildering.

Ideally, before you shop, you should have a pretty good idea of what nutrients you are looking for and in what amounts. You may want to make up a list of the vitamins and minerals you want, based on the strengths and weaknesses of your diet and your needs and preferences. Take the list with you when you go shopping. Then read the ingredients on the labels of a number of different supplements and choose the supplement or supplements that most closely match what you believe are your needs.

Q: That sounds easy enough, but can you give me an example of how that would work?

A: Let's say, for starters, that, like many of the people who take vitamins, you've decided to take a multivitamin and mineral supplement as "insurance" that you are getting enough of all the essential vitamins and minerals. In that case, most experts suggest you buy a multivitamin and mineral supplement that provides 100 percent of the RDA of the nutrients that have an RDA. Most multivitamin and mineral supplements contain some, but not all, of these nutrients, in varying amounts. They tend to provide more of the cheaper and less bulky vitamins, and less of the expensive or bulky ones.

Q: Which nutrients are they missing?

A: You should read labels to find out, since this varies among brands. In general, however, most multivitamin and mineral supplements do not contain phosphorus and iodine, since most Americans get more of these nutrients than they need. On the other hand, studies have shown that people seem to suffer no adverse effects as a result. Also, since vitamin K deficiency is rare, this nutrient is not usually included in a multivitamin. So unless you have some special problem, you probably do not require any of these nutrients as supplements.

Check to see if a supplement contains selenium (not all do), an essential nutrient often lacking in people's diets. Look for one that contains 50 to 200 micrograms (mcg.) of selenium.

Some multivitamin and mineral supplements contain iron. Others do not. High body stores of iron may be linked with an increased risk for heart disease, a study from Finland suggests. So unless you are a premenopausal female, you may not want or need supplemental iron. Check labels to make sure there is none in the supplement you are buying.

Q: What about nutrients that are known to be essential but have no RDA? Should those be in a multivitamin and mineral supplement, too?

A: Instead of an RDA, these nutrients have an **Estimated Safe and Adequate Daily Dietary Intake (ESADDI)**, which is given to essential nutrients for which there is too little information to set an RDA. These nutrients include biotin, pantothenic acid, copper, manganese, fluoride, chromium and molybdenum. A multivitamin and mineral supplement is less likely to contain these nutrients than those with an RDA, and not all experts agree that every one of these nutrients should be in a multivitamin and mineral supplement, says David Roll, Ph.D., professor of medical chemistry in the College of Pharmacy at the University of Utah, in Salt Lake City.

Some experts believe that, of these nutrients, chromium, copper and manganese currently have the strongest research supporting their use as supplements.

Fluoride is not included in most multivitamin and mineral supplements, because, in adults, fluoride supplements have not been proven to be of value, and because high doses cause stomach irritation.

Q: What if I also want to get higher-than-RDA amounts of **antioxidants**, such as vitamins C and E and beta-carotene?

A: Again, check labels. Some multivitamin and mineral supplements do offer high amounts of these nutrients, but most do not. It is easy enough, and sometimes cheaper, to simply purchase single supplements of vitamins C and E and beta-carotene.

Several national brands of multivitamin and mineral supplements are now indicating on their labels that they contain beta-carotene—but they do not state how much beta-carotene actually is in the supplement. If you want to know how much you're getting, find a brand that lists separate amounts of both vitamin A and beta-carotene. Most multiples offer very little beta-carotene—only 1,000 to 2,500 I.U., which is equivalent to 0.5 to 1.5 milligrams of beta-carotene. As a point of comparison, you should know that one inch of carrot contains about 1.5 milligrams of beta-carotene. "[In a multiple-vitamin supplement] you aren't going to get nearly enough to be of significance in terms of an antioxidant effect," Dr. Roll says. Single-nutrient supplements of beta-carotene, on the other hand, often offer 15 milligrams, a bit more than the amount found in one 7½-inch carrot.

Q: I was surprised to learn that the popular multi-vitamin and mineral supplement I was taking contained very little calcium. Is that common?

A: Yes. Most multivitamin and mineral supplements fall short on calcium and also on magnesium. These bulky nutrients just don't fit into a one-a-day pill.

Most multivitamin and mineral supplements contain very little potassium, too, as do single-ingredient potassium supplements. Per tablet, most offer no more than 99 milligrams of potassium, about as much as is found in one inch of banana. The recommended range is 2,000 to 6,000 milligrams of potassium a day. So unless you are taking high-dose potassium supplements prescribed by a doctor, your best bet is to get this mineral from fruits and vegetables and their juices. Wash down your supplement with a cup of orange, grapefruit, carrot or tomato juice for an additional 400 to 500 milligrams of potassium.

Q: I've seen supplements that contain nutrients you haven't even mentioned—choline, PABA, inositol and others. Should I be looking for a supplement that includes these nutrients, too?

A: Most experts feel there is no need for these additional nutrients to be in a supplement, so don't be fooled by a long list of ingredients, which may also include lecithin, glutamic acid, boron, silicon, nickel, vanadium and other nutrients that have not been proven to be necessary in the diets of humans, Dr. Roll says. "These ingredients merely increase the price of a supplement."

Q: What about vitamin formulas just for men or women or for older people? Should I be selecting one of them?

A: Not necessarily. Again, read a product's label to see if it matches your needs. These so-called special formulations do not take the place of a well-balanced multivitamin and mineral supplement, says Dr. Roll. Most contain only two or three nutrients, sometimes in high doses. A premenstrual formula, for instance, may offer many times the RDA of vitamin B6, but contain very little of other B vitamins. An osteoporosis formula may contain calcium but not much of other minerals important for bones.

Q: The health-food store where I shop offers a supplement called "C complex." I've heard of B complex but not C complex. What is it?

A: Formulas labeled C complex usually contain bioflavonoids, substances found in fruits containing vitamin C. They may be listed simply as bioflavonoids or as some of the more commonly used bioflavonoids—**rutin**, **quercetin**, **hesperidin** and **catechin**. None of these compounds is considered essential for health, but several studies suggest the compounds do have activity in the body. They may act as antioxidants, anti-inflammatories and antiviral agents and may also help reduce sensitivity to allergic reactions. Rutin is thought to help reverse capillary fragility, which causes easy bruising and bleeding.

Q: A friend of mine takes a whole handful of vitamin supplements every day. Why would someone do that, rather than simply take a multiple vitamin-mineral tablet?

A: Depends on whom you ask. Some doctors might say a person who uses a large number of single-nutrient vitamin and mineral supplements is simply wasting his money. Others recommend individual supplements of at least some nutrients, especially minerals, because they might be supplied in a form that people with absorption problems can more easily utilize or because the individual nutrients are available in higher doses than a multiple offers.

Q: What about prices? Is expensive better?

A: Not necessarily. Some large national retailers, such as Wal-Mart and K-mart, sell store brands that are similar in formulation to expensive brand-name vitamins, but they cost much less. Again, check labels to see exactly what you are getting for your money. If a manufacturer claims its product is more absorbable or better balanced, you may want to contact the manufacturer and ask for research that backs up such marketing claims.

Q: What's the difference between natural and synthetic vitamins?

A: Natural vitamins are derived from foods. Natural vitamin E, for instance, is isolated from soybean oil. Natural beta-carotene can be derived from carrots or algae. Natural vitamin C can be taken from citrus fruits.

Synthetic vitamins, on the other hand, are constructed from organic molecules found in an array of substances, such as petroleum oil and corn oil. Synthetic vitamins are often used in studies designed to show the health benefits of nutrients in our diet. "Years of testing have established that the natural and synthetic versions of most nutrients are chemically the same," Dr. Roll says. Synthetic vitamins are also much less expensive to make than natural vitamins.

Q: What about vitamin E? I've heard there is a difference between the natural and synthetic versions.

A: It's true that the synthetic version of vitamin E, dl-alpha tocopherol, is different from the natural form, d-alpha tocopherol. The natural form has slightly more biological activity in the body. "This simply means you have to take slightly more synthetic vitamin E to match the effects of the natural version," Dr. Roll says.

Q: Are there natural and synthetic forms of minerals also?

A: No. Minerals are made from materials mined from the ground or otherwise found in nature. Calcium, for instance, is derived from limestone, oyster or egg shells or from naturally occurring beds of calcium carbonate. Minerals may be combined with protein or other ingredients to make them easier to absorb.

Q: Do I have to worry about whether or not the pills I am buying will dissolve properly and be absorbed?

A: You should be concerned, according to experts. They say vitamin makers have addressed the problem of dissolvability but still have a ways to go.

One assurance that the vitamin you are buying will dissolve properly is to look for the letters "U.S.P." on the label. This means the supplement meets manufacturing standards set by the U.S. Pharmacopoeia, an independent, not-for-profit organization that sets standards for strength, quality, purity, packaging and labeling for medical products used in the United States.

Q: What sorts of standards?

A: The first standard states that water-soluble vitamins —C and B vitamins—should disintegrate in an environment that stimulates the digestive tract within 30 minutes if they're uncoated or 45 minutes if coated. Timed-release and chewable supplements aren't covered by these standards, and standards for fat-soluble vitamins and minerals should be ready by 1994. In the meantime, some manufacturers who are already meeting the U.S.P. standards have put the following notice on their labels: "This product is specially formulated to pass a rigid 45-minute laboratory dissolution test."

One helpful hint here about dissolvability and absorption: Usually you can help your body absorb the nutrients in a supplement by taking it at the end of a meal. The digestive juices stimulated by food help the supplement break down and be absorbed.

Q: Can you explain what the amounts used for vitamins and minerals mean? I don't understand the difference between milligrams, micrograms, international units and all the measurement standards you've been using.

A: Fair enough. Here's a quick primer:

• A milligram (abbreviated mg.) is 1/1,000th of a gram; there are 1,000 milligrams in a gram.

• A microgram (abbreviated mcg. or μg.) is 1/1,000th of a milligram; there are 1,000,000 micrograms in a gram.

• There are 28.35 grams in one ounce. (That should give you an idea of how small a gram is.)

• An international unit (I.U.) is an arbitrary unit of measure that has been used for vitamins A and E. However, even though you may continue to see I.U. on vitamin bottles for a while longer, it is no longer the official unit of measure for these vitamins.

Q: How are A and E now measured?

A: The official unit of measure is now **retinol equivalents (RE)** for vitamin A and its various forms (such as beta-carotene) and **tocopherol equivalents (TE)** for vitamin E and its various forms.

Q: But why confuse matters? Why not just use milligrams, like the other vitamins?

A: Researchers have found it necessary to use a unit of measure other than milligrams because vitamins A and E are found in several forms with different levels of activity in the body. These new units of measure make it possible to compare and convert the various forms of these two vitamins, taking into account how active they are.

Q: How can I learn more about what vitamins and minerals I need and in what amounts?

A: The final chapter of this book profiles each essential vitamin and mineral. Note how often you eat foods rich in a particular nutrient to get a feel for whether you're getting enough of that vitamin or mineral.

4 RDAs, RDIs AND ESADDIs

Q: How do I determine how much of a vitamin or mineral I need?

A: Most nutrition experts recommend you start with the RDAs—the Recommended Dietary Allowances.

Q: I have heard of the RDAs and seen them listed for nutrients on cereal boxes. But what are they again?

A: The official definition comes from the Food and Nutrition Board, a committee of nutrition experts at the private, nonprofit National Academy of Sciences. That committee defines the RDAs as "the levels of intake of essential nutrients that, on the basis of scientific knowledge, are judged by the Food and Nutrition Board to be adequate to meet the known nutrient needs of practically all healthy persons."

Q: But what does that mean? Should I make sure I am getting the RDA of every nutrient?

A: As we said, they are generally considered a good place to start. You can compare the amount of a particular nutrient in your diet with the RDA for that nutrient for your sex and age-group. That way you can see if you come out high, low or right on target.

Q: Are the RDAs the same as the **U.S. RDAs?**

A: Not exactly. The Food and Nutrition Board sets different RDAs for people of different ages and sexes. If you look at an RDA chart, you'll find 19 nutrients for 18 different age and sex groups, along with a few more provisional allowances—over 400 values in all.

However, to simplify matters, starting in 1968 the Food and Drug Administration took the highest RDAs—those for teenage boys—and endorsed them as the national standard for everyone, regardless of gender and age, and called them the U.S. RDAs.

Q: So are the U.S.RDAs the numbers used on food and supplement labels?

A: In the past they were. In 1989, however, the Food and Drug Administration (FDA), which plays a role in nutrition labeling for foods, decided to no longer use the RDAs for teenage boys. Instead, they decided to average the RDAs for all the different age-groups and call them **Reference Daily Intakes**, or **RDIs**. Pending regulations mandate that RDIs be used for nutrition labeling of foods. On food labels, the RDI will be listed as the **Daily Value**, or **DV**. Regulations for supplements are also pending.

Q: Why did the FDA decide to revamp the U.S.RDAs?

A: The FDA says the RDIs more accurately target the typical American's nutritional needs. FDA Director John Vanderveen contends that using the old RDAs made the entire population consume more nutrients than it needed.

Q: So does that mean these new values are lower than the old ones?

A: The new figures are considerably lower than those used previously. Switching to this system will slash values on many vitamins and iron by anywhere from 10 to 80 percent. Those heaviest hit: B_{12}, folic acid and vitamin E.

Many nutrition experts are concerned because these recommended amounts are used for many kinds of nutritional support programs and for food fortification. They are afraid that if these reduced figures are implemented, nutritional support programs, such as the National School Lunch and School Breakfast programs and the Nutrition Program for the Elderly, would be downgraded to provide fewer nutrients. That's the reason these regulations are still pending—strong opposition by nutrition researchers has persuaded the FDA to put them on hold for now.

Q: Is this postponement of the RDIs going to affect the new food-labeling requirements I've heard so much about?

A: Not entirely. True, by late 1993 most food labels will have changed. These changes are the result of the Nutrition Labeling and Education Act (NLEA) passed by Congress in October 1992.

The Act intends to standardize food nutrition labeling and make it easier to read. Instead of showing nutrients as a percentage of the U.S.RDA, the new food labels list nutrients as a percentage of Daily Value, or DV, which we mentioned earlier. Unless the FDA-proposed RDIs are adopted, however, the Daily Value will be based on the old U.S.RDAs rather than the RDIs. But "U.S.RDA" will not appear on labels.

Q: Let's get back to the plain, simple RDAs. Do all the vitamins and minerals that are known to be essential have RDAS?

A: No. As we mentioned earlier, for some there is not enough information to come up with an RDA.

Instead, several of these nutrients have Estimated Safe and Adequate Daily Dietary Intakes (ESADDIs), given as a range. These nutrients include biotin, pantothenic acid, copper, manganese, fluoride, chromium and molybdenum.

Some essential nutrients that once had an ESADDI now simply have an estimated minimum requirement. Those nutrients include potassium, sodium and chloride. The Food and Nutrition Board's reason for this change is that they believe under normal circumstances, deficiencies of these nutrients do not exist.

Q: How are RDAs determined?

A: Approximately every five years, a subcommittee of the Food and Nutrition Board reviews the scientific literature on a particular nutrient and comes up with recommendations.

The subcommittee looks at a number of different kinds of studies: those of people on diets containing low or deficient levels of a nutrient, followed by correction of the deficit with measured amounts of the nutrient; studies that measure blood or tissue levels of a nutrient in relation to intake; bio-chemical measurements of tissue saturation or adequacy of molecular function in relation to nutrient intake; studies related to amounts so high that they cause harmful side effects, and other studies.

Q: Sounds like they have good, solid information on which to base their recommendations. Is that the case?

A: It's the ideal, but in reality a lot of information is lacking, which makes the RDAs less accurate than they might be.

Q: What kind of information is lacking?

A: Well, for starters, information is scant on the nutritional requirements for women and children. Most nutrition studies have used young men as subjects, yet the results are applied to women of all ages, children and older men. When it develops its recommendations, the Food and Nutrition Board also considers the results of dietary surveys—questionnaires that ask people what they eat. Unfortunately, dietary surveys are notoriously inaccurate. People simply don't know, don't remember or don't want to remember what it is they eat. So even the best dietary-survey methods are only about 60 percent accurate.

Q: What are RDAs used for?

A: Originally developed during World War II as a way to ensure that military recruits did not suffer from malnutrition, they were quickly adopted as a standard for the general population.

Today they are typically used by meal planners to design menus for groups of captive people—those in the armed services, prisons, hospitals, nursing homes; to interpret food consumption records; to establish standards for food assistance programs such as food stamps, the Supplemental Program for Women, Infants and Children, the National School Lunch and School Breakfast programs, and the Nutrition Program for the Elderly; and as a basis for establishing guidelines for the nutritional labeling of foods and dietary supplements.

Q: You haven't mentioned anything about RDAs and the analysis of an individual's diet. What's the story?

A: The RDAs were not designed to be used to analyze an individual person's diet. In fact, however, "they are used for exactly this purpose simply because they are the best we can offer," says Judi S. Morrill, Ph.D., a professor of nutrition at San Jose State University, in California, and author of *Science, Physiology, and Nutrition: A Primer for the Non-Scientist.*

Dietitians consider that the majority of people, under normal conditions, don't need more than the RDA of a nutrient for normal function, Morrill adds. In fact, not until someone's intake drops below 70 percent of the RDA is it usually considered on the low side.

Q: Why doesn't the Food and Nutrition Board simply lower the RDAs?

A: In fact, they did just that in 1989, for the 10th edition of the RDAs.

Q: Which RDAs were lowered, and by how much?

A: Folic acid, B12, thiamin, riboflavin and niacin were all lowered in some categories. And for women, recommendations were lowered for zinc and iron. For women ages 11 to 50, for instance, the RDA for iron was lowered from 18 to 15 mg.

Also, the range of values for sodium, potassium and chloride were replaced by a minimum requirement, which is appreciably lower than the lower limit previously suggested.

Q: Why were the RDAs lowered?

A: Supposedly, in the words of the Food and Nutrition Board, "the revised RDAs reflect the increasing precision with which certain nutritional needs in the population are known." For instance, in establishing the RDA for the B vitamin folic acid, the Food and Nutrition Board concluded

that "diets containing about half the previous RDA maintain adequate folate status and liver stores."

As a result, it reduced by 50 percent or more for most age-groups the RDA for folic acid, known to play an important role in cell division and protein synthesis. Shortly after the 10th edition of the RDAs was released, several new studies showed that folic-acid deficiency was implicated in neural-tube defects. That information, coming when it did, is not reflected in the current RDAs.

 This sounds strange to me, since all this research now shows that higher amounts for some nutrients can provide important benefits. Am I wrong?

A: No. It seems strange to a lot of nutrition researchers, too. In fact, both the proposed RDIs and the reduced RDAs have churned up a major controversy today in nutrition—the question of *adequate* nutrition versus *optimum* nutrition.

Some nutrition experts agree that most Americans, but certainly not all, are adequately nourished. That is, they do not suffer from the vitamin-deficiency diseases we described earlier, such as scurvy or beriberi, even in milder forms.

On the other hand, new research appears to show that many people do not get optimal amounts of some nutrients— amounts that not only prevent deficiency diseases but also help to protect against chronic diseases, which have only recently been linked with vitamin or mineral intake. These diseases include cancer, heart disease and diabetes, and some doctors contend that the list should include most illnesses. In the words of Dr. Combs, "This new research is challenging old theories and definitions. Today people are looking at longevity and optimum health, which aren't as easy to define or measure."

Q: Do you have any examples of adequate versus optimum amounts?

A: Okay, let's take vitamin E, for example. The RDA for this vitamin is 15 international units, but research suggests additional benefits at much higher amounts—300 I.U. or more.

"No one would say you are going to die if you don't get 300 I.U. of vitamin E per day," says Dr. Combs. "But we think these very high levels may be beneficial and may, in fact, provide a variety of benefits that help ward off chronic diseases and perhaps even slow aging."

Q: Are the RDAs ever going to take this new research into consideration?

A: There's hope yet. The current Food and Nutrition Board does plan to address the question of whether the RDAs should be redefined to include chronic disease in addition to acute deficiency syndromes.

"Defining optimum intake will require reconceptualizing the RDAs and other official information," says Catherine Woteki, Ph.D., R.D., the board's executive director. "We need more specific information to do so. It is a massive task ahead of us."

Q: So where does that leave me now? Am I supposed to use the current RDAs to figure what to eat?

A: For now, consider them the best there is and work with their weaknesses and strengths. You may also want to check the amounts recommended by researchers doing work with a particular nutrient.

Q: Anything else I need to know about the RDAs?

A: Yes. Although they are calculated for people with some special needs, such as pregnant women and nursing mothers, they are not figured to meet the needs of people who are sick or who have trouble absorbing nutrients from their intestines, as would someone with **Crohn's** or **celiac disease**, for instance. Furthermore, the RDAs also may not adequately address the needs of older people.

On the other hand, even the new, lower RDAs go beyond the absolute minimum to prevent deficiency-related diseases. They have a built-in margin of safety. So it's possible you can consistently get less than the RDA for a particular nutrient and suffer no adverse health problems as a result.

5 DIETARY ANALYSIS

Q: Let's say I want to know how much of each vitamin and mineral I am getting in my diet. How do I do that?

A: You can do it the same way a dietitian or nutritionist does it.

Q: Wait a minute—is there a difference between those two nutrition professionals?

A: There are differences in training and certification and, possibly, in orientation to nutrition, all of which we will be happy to explain later. For now, let's continue with the topic of dietary analysis.

Q: Okay, how would a dietitian or nutritionist calculate the vitamins and minerals in my diet?

A: For starters, you will be asked to keep a **food diary**, which lists everything you eat or drink, when you eat it, how much of it you eat and how it is prepared. Is it fried? Steamed? Drenched in garlic butter? Dietitians or nutritionists who counsel people on eating behaviors also ask for additional information: where you ate the food, with whom and your mood at the time. Some ask that you measure food portions; most, however, make do with estimates.

Q: How long am I supposed to keep this diary?

A: A week is ideal. A three-day food diary that includes one weekend day and two weekdays, however, is acceptable. Any time shorter than three days probably wouldn't portray your eating habits accurately.

U.S. DEPARTMENT OF AGRICULTURE'S NUTRIENT DATABASE

Q: What happens to the diary?

A: The dietitian or nutritionist analyzes it, in many cases using one of several computer programs. These programs include thousands of foods, broken down into their components, including the amounts of vitamins and minerals in each. As the information in your food diary goes into the program, the computer breaks down the nutrients in your diet, including vitamins and minerals, calories, protein, fats and carbohydrates.

Q: That sounds too easy to be true. Is it accurate?

A: Glad you asked. Most of the computer programs are based on the U.S. Department of Agriculture's Nutrient Database, probably the most complete source of nutritional information in the world. So, it's about as accurate as dietary assessment gets these days, given that there are problems with any kind of dietary analysis.

Q: Like what?

A: For one thing, missing data. It might be easy to figure out someone's calcium or iron intake, but when it comes to chromium, copper or vitamin K, the numbers just aren't in the Nutrient Database for many foods, or the numbers may not be considered accurate. Currently, there's no way to know for sure what someone's intake is for some nutrients, especially for trace minerals.

Data are also more likely to be missing for processed foods than for whole foods. So if you eat a lot of frozen dinners and fudge pops, for example, it may be harder to calculate your intake of individual nutrients than if you were eating oatmeal, apples and chicken.

Q: Any other problems?

A: **Bioavailability**, or how well you absorb a nutrient, varies tremendously in foods and is not always taken into account. Although cooking methods are taken into consideration in these calculations, cooking times or the freshness of foods is not. Such factors influence the amount of vitamins and minerals in a food, with some nutrients much more sensitive to these factors than others. Folic acid, for instance, found in leafy greens, may be reduced by as much as one-third by cooking. Potassium also is leached out of vegetables in cooking water.

Q: Let's say I want to use the USDA Nutrient Database or a nutritional analysis computer program. How do I do that?

A: You may be allowed to use the USDA Nutrient Database at the nearest college with a nutrition department. Another possibility is for a college nutrition department to allow you access to a computer software program that does dietary analysis. You may also wish to purchase the USDA Nutrient Database, or a software program based on the USDA Nutrient Database. Such software programs are often advertised in nutrition journals, such as the *Journal of the American Dietetic Association.* However, they are expensive. One of the more popular programs, Nutritionist 5, costs around $600.

Q: What if I don't have access to a computer?

A: The same nutritional breakdown of foods is available in a series of USDA handbooks, called *Composition of Foods.* The most recent series, number 8, includes 22 volumes, which cover thousands of foods: dairy and egg products, spices and herbs, baby foods, fats and oils, poultry products, soups, sauces and gravies, sausage and luncheon meats, breakfast cereals, fruits and fruit juices, pork products, vegetables and vegetable products, beef products and others. Consult your public library or a nearby college library.

Q: I've heard that I can have my diet computer-analyzed by mail. Is that true? How's it done? Is it accurate? Expensive?

A: Yes, it is possible to have your diet computer-analyzed by mail. Several companies, including some nutritional testing laboratories, offer the service.

You first fill out what's called a food-frequency survey. This looks like a long multiple-choice test, includes many foods and beverages, and asks you to mark how often you eat each food or drink each beverage. Surveys vary, but most allow you to mark how many times a day, week or month you consume something like, say, oatmeal or black olives.

The survey results are analyzed via computer the same way a dietitian or nutritionist might analyze a food diary. The results are sent to you in a computer printout that may show your midpoint and range for each nutrient and what percentage above or below the RDA you are.

Q: Is that all these analyses do?

A: Some analyses also show you how varied your diet is among the food groups. For instance, the analysis may show you approximately how many servings per day, on average, you are eating of dairy foods, meats and grains and compare your intake with dietary guidelines to let you know whether your diet exceeds or falls short of the guidelines. Many of the surveys also send along a "Diet Discussion" or some other printed material that explains the significance of your findings and provides suggestions for improvement, such as cutting back or adding particular foods or food groups to your diet.

DIETITIANS AND NUTRITIONISTS

Q: How different are such surveys from the kind that might be done professionally?

A: These surveys are similar to what a dietitian or nutritionist might offer and are the same sort that are used in research, says Mona Sutnick, R.D., a dietitian in private practice and a spokesperson for the American Dietetic Association. "They are considered fairly accurate, as long as the information you put in them is accurate."

But these surveys suffer the same problems that other forms of dietary assessment have. They may be missing values for some foods, especially processed foods, and for some nutrients, especially trace minerals.

Q: Is it necessary to consult a professional to make best use of a dietary analysis?

A: Unless you have some knowledge of nutrition, even with the interpretive printout, it may be difficult for you to figure out what the results mean for you, Sutnick contends. "This is where professional guidance may be useful," she says.

A dietitian or nutritionist (or even the rare nutritionally knowledgeable doctor, who knows your medical condition and history and your health concerns and who may have the results of blood tests on hand) can help you figure out what your computerized dietary assessment really means and the best changes you can make as a result of its findings.

Q: How do I know who to choose—a dietitian, nutritionist or doctor?

A: Any one of them may be able to help you. Actually, a doctor is more likely to refer you to a dietitian or nutritionist than do nutritional counseling himself and, in fact, that's probably the best thing for most doctors to do. Their knowledge of nutrition is usually quite limited. We have more to say on doctors and nutrition in the next chapter.

Q: What if I am choosing between a dietitian and a nutritionist? Can you return to my earlier question on the differences between the two?

A: Anyone can call herself a nutritionist, whether or not she has special training in nutrition. On the other hand, only people who have been certified in dietetics by the American Dietetic Association (ADA) can call themselves registered dietitians (R.D., for short). It's a sort of trademark that no one else can use.

According to the ADA, to be a registered dietitian a person must have a bachelor's degree in foods and nutrition or dietetics from an accredited college or university; complete a work-study program or internship (usually lasting 12 months or more and always ADA-approved) to gain practical experience; pass a national qualifying examination administered by the ADA; and maintain the R.D. status through continuing-education courses.

Q: Does this mean I should choose an R.D. as my nutritionist?

A: Not necessarily. They are valid sources of information from their perspective, but many authorities in the field contend that the R.D.'s perspective is outdated—too focused on the four basic food groups and food management rather than more timely issues, such as supplementation and preventive medicine.

So don't accept at face value any person's credentials without asking a lot of questions.

Q: Where can I get a list of R.D.'s?

A: You can get the names and phone numbers of three registered dietitians closest to you by calling the American Dietetic Association's referral service. That toll-free number is (800) 366-1655 (10 a.m. to 5 p.m. Eastern time). Be prepared to furnish your ZIP code.

And now, on to doctors, the other professionals whom you may wish to consult.

6 FINDING A DOCTOR KNOWLEDGEABLE IN NUTRITION

Q: My experience has been that most doctors either aren't interested in nutrition or that they know less about it than I do. Is this a common finding?

A: It certainly seems to be a common complaint among patients seeing traditional doctors. "For about 50 years now, people have been complaining that their doctors know little or nothing about nutrition, and just about everyone agrees that the problem continues to persist," says Kathy Kolasa, Ph.D., a professor of nutrition in the department of family medicine at East Carolina University, Greenville, North Carolina.

In fact, a recent survey of nutrition-related practices among M.D.'s painted a discouraging picture. For starters, only about 11 percent of the 30,000 doctors to whom surveys were mailed responded. It's true that the majority of those who did reply agreed with positive statements about nutrition, such as: "Diet has an important role in disease prevention"; "In many cases, medication could be reduced or eliminated if patients followed a recommended diet"; and "Doctors should spend more time exploring dietary habits during patient evaluation."

Q: So what's the problem?

A: The problem is that, when it comes to putting those attitudes into practice, most doctors fall far short, according to this survey, which was conducted by researchers at Tufts University School of Medicine. For example, only about two-thirds of doctors said they routinely attempt to identify patients with nutritional problems. And only one-third said they regularly use recent nutrition-related research results to improve their patients' care. When they do prescribe healthful diets, only 20 percent keep in mind lifestyle factors that affect their patients' eating habits, such as cultural food preferences and economic status. And only about 20 percent suggest counseling with registered dietitians or nutritionists or refer patients to organizations that can provide nutrition information.

Q: Why are so many doctors lacking when it comes to nutrition?

A: For starters, their educations placed little or no emphasis on nutrition, despite the fact that 6 of the nation's 10 leading causes of death are inextricably linked to our diets: heart disease, cerebrovascular disease, cancer, type-II diabetes, arteriosclerosis and alcohol-induced cirrhosis of the liver.

"Nutrition education programs in U.S. medical schools are largely inadequate to meet the present and future demands of the medical profession," according to a report by the National Research Council's Committee on Nutrition in Medical Education. That 1985 report found that, while most schools teach nutrition in some form or another, only one in five teaches it as a separate, required course. Therefore, in the vast majority of schools, nutrition is relegated to the sort of hit-or-miss approach that often is characteristic of elective courses.

Q: Are there any doctors who are knowledgeable in nutrition? How can I find one who is?

A: They're there, but they're rare. Shop the same way you would for any new doctor, but add questions that specifically address the topic of nutrition.

Believe it or not, asking around is considered one of the best ways to come up with names of doctors you may want to contact. In addition to asking friends and relatives, contact nutritionists and dietitians in your area to find out what doctors they work with and recommend.

You may be lucky enough to live near a medical school that has a department of preventive medicine or, rarer still, a nutrition department. If so, you may be able to find a doctor who is associated with either of those departments and who incorporates sound nutrition into her practice, when appropriate.

Q: Any other good shopping tips?

A: People associated with a local branch of the Arthritis Foundation or American Heart Association, or with health clubs, diet centers or even health-foods stores, may be able to provide you with leads.

Q: What kinds of questions should I ask?

A: Call the doctors' offices, explain that you are a potential patient, and ask the following questions:
• I am looking for a doctor who is knowledgeable in nutrition. Does the doctor provide nutritional counseling to her patients?
• For what kinds of health problems does she provide nutritional counseling? Weight loss? Heart disease? Diabetes? Chronic fatigue syndrome? Depression?
• Does the doctor refer patients on a regular basis to a nutritionist or dietitian? ("A doctor who makes regular referrals to a nutritionist or dietitian is likely to appreciate the importance of nutrition," Dr. Kolasa points out. "If a doctor says she does not refer to a nutritionist or dietitian, you know she isn't paying attention to the nutritional needs of her patients.")
• Is the doctor board-certified in nutrition? If not, does she have any special training in nutrition? How long did she train, and where?
• Is she affiliated with a university?

• Is she a member of any nutrition-related organizations? Which ones?

• Does the doctor sell supplements from her office? (It's true that some people don't like doctors who push vitamin supplements, but "this isn't the big no-no it was just a few years ago," Dr. Kolasa contends.)

Q: **Is there a particular medical specialist who is most likely to know a lot about nutrition?**

A: A doctor in any specialty could fit the bill. But in traditional, or **allopathic**, medicine, only doctors specializing in family medicine are required to take nutrition courses as part of their residency training after medical school. **Internists**, obstetricians and gynecologists, along with other specialists, may take nutrition courses as electives, but their specialties do not require such courses.

The Tufts University survey found that doctors who change their own diets tend to express the most positive attitudes about nutrition and are more likely to translate those attitudes into diet-related patient care. The survey also found that graduates of foreign medical schools, doctors affiliated with universities, and doctors younger than age 45 tended to express more of an interest in nutrition than other doctors.

Q: **I know that doctors can take special training that allows them to be board-certified in specialties like gynecology or cardiology. Can a doctor be board-certified in nutrition?**

A: Yes. Currently, a doctor can be certified in nutrition by the American Board of Nutrition, which establishes standards for qualification of people as specialists in the field of human and clinical nutrition, and which administers examinations. To qualify for certification by the American Board of Nutrition, a person must hold either an M.D. or Ph.D. in a related field, such as clinical nutrition or preventive medicine. He must also pass the examination given by the board. Currently, about 400 doctors or researchers are certified by the American Board of Nutrition.

To find out if a particular doctor is certified by this organization, you can call or write to the American Board of Nutrition, 9650 Rockville Pike, Bethesda, MD 20815; or call (301) 530-7110.

Note that this certification is not approved by the American Board of Medical Specialties, a Chicago-based independent regulatory board that has established certification standards for 24 medical specialties. Currently, the American Board of Nutrition is developing a certification program designed to gain the approval of the American Board of Medical Specialties.

Q: **What about other professional certifications or memberships in professional organizations? What do such memberships say about a doctor's expertise?**

A: Some organizations offer memberships based on education and expertise; others, however, admit anyone who can pay the membership fees.

A doctor may belong to a group active in the clinical application of nutrition, research and education, including continuing nutrition education for doctors. Groups that offer membership based on education and expertise include the American Society for Clinical Nutrition, the American Institute of Nutrition and the American College of Nutrition.

There are many other nutrition-oriented institutes, societies and foundations to which a doctor can belong. If your doctor cites membership in a particular organization as proof of his expertise, ask him about the requirements for membership in that organization: Does it require an advanced degree? Leading research? Outstanding clinical performance? Or simply a membership fee?

Q: What about **osteopathic** doctors? Do they know more about nutrition than regular doctors?

A: Opinion seems to be that they do, but there are no studies to prove that they are any better trained in nutrition or that they are more likely than allopathic doctors to incorporate nutrition into their practices.

Q: Wait a minute—exactly what is an osteopathic doctor? How is such a doctor different from an allopathic one?

A: An osteopathic doctor—or doctor of osteopathy (D.O.)—is trained in the branch of medicine known as osteopathy, which holds the philosophy that the body is an interrelated system. For this reason, osteopaths tend to be more holistic in their approach to care, using hands-on diagnostic techniques instead of or in addition to laboratory tests, and offering other treatments besides drugs and surgery (most notably manipulation of bones, muscles and joints of the body). For the most part, however, their medical training and licensing are the same as those of M.D.'s. There are only about 28,000 osteopathic doctors in the United States, compared to about 500,000 allopathic doctors.

For more information about this branch of medicine, contact the American Osteopathic Association, 142 East Ontario St., Chicago, IL 60611; or call (312) 280-5800.

Q: Who else might offer nutrition counseling?

A: Both **homeopathic** and **naturopathic** doctors may offer nutrition counseling. But don't assume that because a doctor is less drug-oriented—as homeopaths and naturopaths usually are—that she is more nutritionally focused, or that she is any better trained in nutrition than a traditional doctor.

Q: What is homeopathic medicine?

A: Homeopathic medicine holds that "like cures like" and that medicines that cause symptoms of diseases in healthy people bring about cures in sick people. Another basic tenet of homeopathy is that a whole person must be treated and not just the disease—and it is here that a person's diet and nutritional status may be taken into account.

For more information on this branch of medicine, contact the National Center for Homeopathy, Suite 306, 801 North Fairfax St., Alexandria, Virginia 22314; or call (703) 548-7790.

Q: And naturopathic medicine?

A: Naturopathic medicine is a healing art that emphasizes the body's natural healing forces. It is a drugless therapy that makes use of massage, light, heat, air and water.

To a naturopath, a person's medical history is the most important piece of information used to make a diagnosis, although he also relies on lab tests and other diagnostic techniques, such as x-rays, scans, physical examinations and so on.

Q: So where does nutritional counseling come in?

A: Naturopaths consider diet and nutrition essential to good health, and advise people on proper nutrition, including what to eat and what to avoid. In some cases, depending upon the patient's condition or complaint, naturopaths recommend fasting as one method for detoxifying the body before beginning a new regimen of diet and nutrition.

For more information on naturopathy, contact the American Association of Naturopathic Physicians, P.O. Box 20386, Seattle, WA 98102; or call (206) 323-7610.

Q: What if I like my current doctor, but she doesn't know enough about nutrition to suit me?

A: Tell her! As a health-care consumer, you have the ability to influence what doctors offer by demanding what you want. Your doctor may be willing to take additional education in nutrition or to begin referrals to a dietitian or nutritionist if she realizes that is what her patients want.

So ask questions. What can I do to avoid osteoporosis? How can I change my diet to help my arthritis? What vitamins can I take to reduce my risks of heart disease?

Q: But aren't there tests my doctor can do to help assess my nutritional status?

A: So glad you asked. We have a lot to say about that in the next chapter.

7 TESTS TO ASSESS VITAMIN AND MINERAL STATUS

Q: I remember from Chapter 5 that a dietary analysis can help me determine my nutritional status, but there must be other ways. Can a physical examination or tests allow a doctor to determine how I am absorbing and utilizing nutrients in my body?

A: Yes. A doctor can use a number of methods to determine your nutritional status. He should start with a detailed medical history and a careful physical examination that includes checking your height and weight; the condition of your skin, hair and fingernails; mucous membranes inside your mouth and eyes; your tongue and gums. All these body parts can provide clues to your health.

Q: Clues? Like what?

A: A bright red tongue, for instance, might be a sign of riboflavin or iron deficiency. Skin that feels like coarse sandpaper, a condition called follicular hyperkeratosis, could indicate a vitamin A, E or B-complex deficiency. Cracks around the corners of your mouth could mean you're low on riboflavin. And spoon-shaped fingernails could mean your iron levels are hitting rock-bottom.

Q: Must I be severely deficient in a nutrient for signs of deficiency to be so apparent?

A: Not necessarily. A good history and a physical exam, if done by someone trained to do examinations for borderline nutritional insufficiencies, can provide important clues toward diagnosis, experts say. But don't count on just any doctor to "eyeball" your nutritional status, warns Howerde Sauberlich, M.D., director of the division of experimental nutrition at the University of Alabama in Birmingham. "The average physician is not familiar with these sorts of symptoms and will not pick up on them," he says.

Doctors who have incorporated nutrition into their practices, though, rely on those "eyeball" observations, along with dietary analysis, medical history and certain tests to make their diagnosis.

Q: What kinds of laboratory tests might a doctor do during a nutritional assessment?

A: That depends, in part, on what he finds during other aspects of the examination. Many different types of tests are available—blood and urine, as well as hair and even saliva. These tests are diverse and can be confusing to doctors as well as patients. Even experts don't always agree on which test best measures a particular nutrient or what the results of a test mean. And sometimes a doctor orders a test not because it is the most accurate to measure a person's status for a particular nutrient, but because it is the only test readily available.

BLOOD TESTS

Q: What can you tell me about blood tests to assess vitamin or mineral status?

A: These tests measure vitamins or minerals in serum (or plasma), the clear fluid that separates from blood on clotting; in cells found in the blood, such as red or white blood cells; or in whole blood, which includes serum and cells, along with any particles found in blood.

Blood tests can be categorized into two basic groups— screening tests and so-called functional tests. Screening tests measure directly the amount of a vitamin or mineral in blood. They can detect severe deficiencies but they often overlook less severe deficiencies that may nevertheless cause physical or mental symptoms. Screening tests are often the only kind of test that a traditional doctor orders, if he orders any nutritional tests at all.

Q: What are functional tests?

A: Functional tests are considered to be more sensitive to borderline nutritional deficiencies than screening tests are. These tests assess vitamin or mineral levels indirectly, by measuring enzyme activity or metabolic activity in cells associated with a vitamin or mineral.

Q: Can you give me some examples of the types of blood tests you are talking about?

A: Iron is a good example because it is frequently and accurately measured. Iron status can be measured in a number of ways, and most doctors believe that using several measures provides a more accurate assessment of iron status than any single measure.

The first (and easiest) tests usually performed are: **hemoglobin**, which measures the amount of iron in red blood cells, and hematocrit, which simply indicates the ratio of red cells to serum. If these prove to be low, a doctor can then do three more tests to determine the cause of a deficiency: a total iron test, which measures all the iron circulating in someone's blood; a serum ferritin test, which measures the body's storage form of iron and can detect if the body has been dipping into its iron stores; and a serum transferrin, or total iron binding capacity test, which measures a protein used to transport iron from the liver or elsewhere in the body to wherever it's needed.

Q: Are other minerals measured this precisely?

A: No. Many of the standard tests used to measure other minerals frequently are not very sensitive to changes in body status.

Take zinc, for example. Body levels of this mineral can be measured several ways, including plasma levels and levels in red or white blood cells. "But zinc researchers at a recent conference concluded that there is no one satisfactory way to measure zinc status," according to Dr. Sauberlich. "Plasma zinc is the easiest and most available, but with this test, it is hard to identify someone who is not severely deficient. Someone only moderately deficient in zinc would have normal results with this test. And the red- or white-blood-cell tests for zinc all have problems, too."

Q: Any other nutrients?

A: Calcium and magnesium are often measured using a serum level, but many nutrition-oriented doctors consider serum a poor way to measure calcium or magnesium status, since the body carefully regulates serum levels of both calcium and magnesium, robbing bones of calcium if necessary to maintain adequate blood levels.

One study showed that serum levels of magnesium can be normal even when tissue stores of magnesium are so depleted as to cause heart arrhythmias.

Q: Are the tests for vitamins any more sensitive to small changes in body status than most of the tests for minerals?

A: Some are and some aren't. As with minerals, it depends on the test. Functional tests are considered to be more accurate than general screening tests.

Q: It sounds like I can't always rely on a laboratory test to tell me what's going on in my body nutrition-wise. Is that the case?

A: Unfortunately, it is. That's why most doctors rely on a number of diagnostic findings, including laboratory tests, to determine your nutritional status.

URINE TESTS

Q: What about urine tests? What can they tell me about my nutritional status?

A: Urine contains waste matter filtered out of blood by the kidneys. One liter of urine can be thought of as the end result of more than 1,000 liters of blood passing through the kidneys.

Urine is most often tested for sugar, or glucose. A high level of glucose in urine could mean diabetes. Protein levels are also measured. High amounts of protein can indicate kidney problems. These tests, however, do not indicate vitamin or mineral status.

Q: What urine tests do measure vitamins and minerals?

A: Less commonly, urine is tested for the by-products, or metabolites, of certain vitamins. Abnormalities could mean a problem with the body's metabolism, which is its ability to burn carbohydrates or fats. Abnormal levels of metabolites in the urine may be related to vitamin deficiencies.

Urine can also be tested for its levels of minerals, such as calcium or potassium. But these tests are usually done only in research settings.

Other urine tests can be done that give some indication of a person's nutritional status, exposure to toxic metals and metabolism. Many of these tests, however, are less sensitive than blood tests and so may be used only to corroborate the findings of blood tests.

HAIR ANALYSIS

Q: Can hair analysis tell me anything about my nutritional status?

A: Most nutrition professionals do not consider hair a good indicator of nutritional status. One reason is that hair growth tends to slow down in people who are truly malnourished, increasing mineral concentrations in hair while body stores drop. Hair can also be contaminated by shampoo, dyes or even by the metal of the scissors used to cut it.

Q: So doctors, even those specializing in nutrition, don't order this sort of test?

A: Some continue to use hair analysis and consider it helpful. Hair, in fact, can be an indicator of exposure to heavy metals over a period of time—specifically, exposure to arsenic, lead, mercury, cadmium and aluminum.

Q: When would it be considered appropriate to test for heavy-metal exposure?

A: The answer to that may depend on your practitioner. Some doctors believe many people today risk exposure to potential toxins through air, water or soil pollution, lead-soldered copper pipes, or pesticides and herbicides. Others believe the only people at high enough risk to warrant testing are those with known exposures, such as might occur through jobs, accidental spills or contaminated wells.

Q: What does a doctor do with the results of a hair analysis?

A: Even though hair analysis itself is up for debate— whether or not to do it—the nutrition experts do agree on one issue: Any hair-analysis findings concerning vitamin and mineral deficiencies or toxicities need to be confirmed with other tests (blood tests, for example) before any treatment recommendations can be made.

SALIVA TESTS

Q: When would saliva be tested?

A: Saliva testing is not a standard test but it is used by some researchers to check zinc, copper and magnesium status, says Robert I. Henkin, M.D., Ph.D., director of the taste and smell clinic at the Center for Molecular Nutrition and Sensory Disorders at Georgetown University Medical Center, in Washington, D.C.

In checking a person's zinc status, for instance, saliva is tested for its level of gustin, a zinc-dependent enzyme that influences taste-bud growth, Dr. Henkin says. Gustin levels drop off when someone is deficient in zinc. Gustin levels also may drop if someone has an abnormality of zinc metabolism, a problem that is difficult to measure any other way, Dr. Henkin says. "We do this test, and so do a few other centers. It is not considered strictly a research method."

Q: It sounds like there is a good chance my doctor will order a test that doesn't do me much good or, worse, that provides misinformation. Is there?

A: It all depends on the doctor and why she wants to do a particular test.

Undoubtedly, you want to be assured that your doctor is ordering tests in a logical, progressive manner. And that's why it is always a good idea to ask her some questions about any test she orders: Why are you ordering this test? What do you expect to find? How accurate is this test? What do you plan to do with the results of this test? What is the potential that I will be misdiagnosed or mistreated as a result of this test? What does it cost? Will I be paying for it myself, or will my health insurance cover it? What happens if I don't have this test? Will we be missing a potentially essential piece of information regarding my diagnosis? Will it change my course of treatment?

Ask for a copy of the test results to read as you review the findings with your doctor. Ask what the test means in terms of your condition, or in terms of risk factors for disease.

8 VITAMINS

VITAMIN A AND BETA-CAROTENE

Q: What is vitamin A?

A: Vitamin A is a clear yellow oil and one of the four fat-soluble vitamins, along with vitamins D, E and K. That means it dissolves in organic solvents, such as ether or cleaning fluid, and, in the body, is absorbed and transported in a manner similar to that of fats. If you have problems absorbing fat in your intestines, you run a higher-than-normal risk of developing a vitamin A deficiency.

Q: If vitamin A is fat-soluble, does that mean it's found in foods that contain fat?

A: Yes. Vitamin A occurs naturally only in foods of animal origin, such as liver, which is the storage place for vitamin A in animals and humans; some seafood; butter; whole milk and egg yolks. This form of vitamin A is usually called preformed vitamin A, or **retinol**. Retinol is also added to skim and low-fat milk. A particularly rich source of vitamin A, cod-liver oil, is sometimes used to make vitamin A supplements.

Q: But isn't vitamin A found in carrots? Carrots don't contain much fat.

A: Good question. Carrots don't actually contain vitamin A, but carrots and other orange and yellow vegetables and fruits and dark green leafy vegetables contain certain substances, called **carotenoids**, that the body can convert to vitamin A.

Carotenoids are said to be **provitamins**, or to have provitamin A activity. The best known of these provitamins is beta-carotene, which does not necessarily have the most vitamin A activity of any carotenoid but which is abundant in many foods.

Q: What's the RDA for vitamin A?

A: It's 1,000 RE, or retinol equivalents (5,000 I.U.), for men, and 800 RE (4,000 I.U.) for women.

Q: Again, what is a retinol equivalent?

A: It's an arbitrary unit of measurement that allows the different forms of vitamin A, all with varying levels of biological activity in the body, to be compared and measured. One retinol equivalent equals 1 microgram of retinol or 6 micrograms of beta-carotene.

Q: How much vitamin A do people actually get?

A: Surveys show that, in general, people seem to get enough vitamin A, although they are getting most of it as preformed vitamin A, not beta-carotene. According to one study, the average intake is 5,440 I.U. a day.

Q: Are there problems with toxicity? What are they?

A: Because it is fat-soluble and can be stored in the liver for long periods of time, vitamin A is considered to

have a fairly high potential for toxicity. Before signs of toxicity begin to appear in most adults, it appears necessary to
take a single large dose (in supplement form) of 250,000 to
300,000 I.U., or smaller amounts of 50,000 I.U. or so for
long periods of time.

However, some individuals appear to display some symptoms of toxicity at daily doses as low as 25,000 I.U. Those
signs include bone and joint pain, hair loss, skin dryness,
itching and flaking, weakness and fatigue, and may also include other symptoms, such as headache and vision problems.
Stopping the excessive dosage usually reverses symptoms
with no permanent damage.

Q: Is beta-carotene also toxic in large amounts?

A: No, beta-carotene has no toxicity problems, even at
extremely high levels, whether it's gotten from foods
or supplements.

Q: What exactly does vitamin A do?

A: Vitamin A is essential for human health. A deficiency
may cause night blindness and other eye disorders,
lowered resistance to infection, poor tooth development, a
stunting of growth and fertility problems.

Vitamin A deficiency also causes weakening of epithelial
cells, which cover the internal and external surfaces of the
body, including the lining of blood vessels and other small
cavities. Epithelial cells can be found in the skin, lungs,
developing teeth, inner ear, cornea, gonads, glands and their
ducts, gums, the front of the lens of the eye, the sensory part
of the nose, the cervix and other areas of the body. Vitamin A
must be present for these cells to differentiate—to go from
their immature to their mature states. If these cells fail to
mature because of a vitamin A deficiency, often the result is
an alteration in skin and mucous membranes that resembles a
precancerous condition, and that, given the proper condi-

tions, can lead to cancer. Weakened epithelial tissues also pave the way for a variety of infections.

Q: How would I know if I'm low in vitamin A?

A: Signs of vitamin A deficiency include night blindness, or impaired adaptation of the eyes to darkness; a lack of normal mucous secretion, including dry eyes and mouth; susceptibility to infection, such as sinus trouble or sore throats; xerophthalmia, an eye condition characterized by swollen lids and sticky discharge from the eyes; and a condition called follicular hyperkeratosis, where the skin feels like coarse sandpaper. Recent studies have even found hearing disorders in vitamin A-deficient people.

Q: Does beta-carotene do anything that's different from vitamin A?

A: Even though beta-carotene itself is not considered a vitamin, it does seem to have activity in the body independent of its conversion to vitamin A, and much of that activity seems to revolve around cancer prevention and protection against heart disease. That's why researchers now distinguish beta-carotene from preformed vitamin A.

Q: How did researchers figure out that there is a difference between the two?

A: Studies done over the years seem to indicate that people who get lots of vitamin A from plants, as carotenoids, are at less risk of developing cancer of the lungs, cervix and gastrointestinal tract, while people who get most of their vitamin A from animal foods are not protected. In animal studies, beta-carotene has provided protection against chemical- or radiation-induced cancer. And in human studies, it also seems to offer some cancer protection.

Q: What about heart disease and beta-carotene?

A: Several recent studies also indicate that beta-carotene provides some protection against heart disease.
One, the Physicians' Health Study, a long-term study involving 22,000 male doctors, found that among 333 men who already had evidence of cardiovascular disease, those taking beta-carotene supplements over six years had half as many strokes, heart attacks, sudden cardiac deaths or surgeries to open or bypass clogged coronary arteries as those taking placebos. In the study, the doctors took 50 milligrams of beta-carotene every other day (equivalent to 83,720 I.U.).

Q: Any studies on women?

A: So glad you asked. A large study of nurses, by the same researchers, found a 22 percent reduction in the risk of heart attack and a 40 percent reduction in stroke risk for women with high intakes of fruits and vegetables rich in beta-carotene, compared with women whose intakes were low. The low beta-carotene group was getting fewer than 6 milligrams of carotene a day, the amount found in less than half a carrot. The high intake group was getting more than 15 to 20 milligrams a day—one to two on the carrot scale. So the difference between the two groups was only about 10 to 15 milligrams, about the amount found in a single serving of a beta-carotene-rich fruit or vegetable.

Q: How does beta-carotene provide cancer and heart-disease protection?

A: Like vitamins C and E, beta-carotene works as an antioxidant, but in its own unique way.

Q: Hold on a minute. I know you explained this previously, but I need a refresher. What exactly is an antioxidant?

A: An antioxidant is a molecule that helps limit an oxidative reaction by neutralizing free radicals.

Q: What's that again?

A: Oxidative reactions—reactions that involve oxygen— take place all the time in our bodies. They, for instance, help our bodies generate energy. Oxidative reactions also turn butter rancid, coat iron fences with rust, and turn a slice of apple brown.

While necessary in the body, oxidative reactions are potentially harmful. The reactions form highly reactive, molecularly unbalanced substances called free radicals. Free radicals lack electrons and attempt to steal electrons from other molecules to regain their balance. A victimized molecule itself becomes a free radical, initiating a chain reaction of multiplying free radicals that oxidize a large amount of cells very quickly.

Q: Are you saying that oxidative chain reactions can harm cells?

A: Yes, oxidative reactions can damage the fatty outer membranes of cells, impairing the ability of molecules to move in and out of cells, explains Jeffrey Blumberg, Ph.D., chief of the antioxidants research laboratory at the USDA Human Nutrition Research Center on Aging at Tufts University, Boston. "It means the cell may not work right or, if the damage is bad enough, the cell may die."

Free radicals that get inside a cell can damage the cell's genetic material, DNA, causing mutations that have the potential to lead to cancer. Free radicals can also damage a cell's energy source, the mitochondria, destroying the cell's ability to produce the energy it needs to function, Dr. Blumberg says.

Q: So antioxidants like beta-carotene and vitamins E and C help to limit oxidative chain reactions?

A: Yes. Antioxidants help stop these chain reactions by offering up one of their electrons to free radicals and, thus, neutralizing them. The antioxidants do not become free radicals themselves. Instead, they simply become inactive.

Q: Okay. So beta-carotene and vitamins E and C help limit the cell damage that can be caused by oxidative reactions. But what does this mean in terms of health and disease prevention?

A: It means that anywhere in the body that oxidative reactions are contributing to a disease process, these nutrients might help prevent or limit that disease.

Q: Can you give me some examples?

A: Take eyes, for instance. The lenses of the eyes are exposed to oxidative damage from sunlight. This oxidative damage can lead to cataracts, a condition where the normally clear lens of an eye becomes milky white and opaque. Worldwide in incidence, cataracts are one of the most common causes of blindness among older people. In both animal and human studies, antioxidant nutrients help prevent cataracts. They work by protecting proteins in the lens from oxidative damage from sunlight. In one study, extra amounts of either vitamin E or vitamin C reduced the incidence of cataracts by about 30 percent.

Lungs are also vulnerable to oxidative damage from pollutants in the air, such as ozone and nitrogen dioxide. Animal studies indicate that low levels of vitamin E and other antioxidants increase pollutant damage to the lungs, and that high levels of vitamins E and C and beta-carotene help protect lungs.

Q: It sounds like there is really strong evidence that this stuff protects against cancer. Is that right?

A: Let's say that researchers are excited, but until they get results of several clinical trials currently in progress, the case won't be sewn up. Two studies found no apparent association, and one of those studies, by well-known researcher Walter Willett of Harvard University, found no association between blood levels of carotenoids and five-year risk of cancer.

Still, researchers suggest you eat plenty of fruits and vegetables, and include those containing beta-carotene. Population studies do show the benefits of eating at least five servings a day of fruits and vegetables, even if research has yet to determine conclusively whether it's the beta-carotene in the foods or some other component that's offering protection.

Q: Are any other carotenoids thought to help protect against cancer?

A: Yes. Other carotenoids besides beta-carotene are known to act as antioxidants, although they are still much less studied than beta-carotene. Exactly how they offer protection is unknown.

These carotenoids include lutein, zeaxanthin, beta-cryptoxanthin, lycopene, alpha carotene and others. Studies of cells in culture and with animals demonstrate that these carotenoids can protect against cancer.

Q: Does the substance called retinol, which you earlier called preformed vitamin A, play any role in cancer prevention?

A: Most of the dietary studies that have looked for an association between retinol and cancer have not found an association.

One study found that people whose diets were high in some retinol-containing foods seemed to have an increased risk for cancer, but it seems more likely that the association was due to the high fat content of the foods—eggs, butter, sour cream—than to the vitamin A content.

Q: Aren't some acne drugs made from vitamin A? I heard they were also being used to treat cancer. Are they?

A: There are two types of acne drugs made from derivatives of vitamin A. Both have similar structures. One is Retin-A (tretinoin), a topically applied gel used for the treatment of acne, wrinkles and a potentially precancerous skin condition called actinic keratosis.

The other drug is Accutane (isotretinoin), a drug taken orally in the form of soft gelatin capsules. Accutane is used for the treatment of severe acne.

Accutane—but not Retin-A—has been used experimentally to reverse potentially precancerous changes in the cells lining the inside of the mouth, a condition called oral leukoplakia. About 8 percent of Americans, mostly smokers, develop this condition. Approximately 5 to 15 percent go on to develop oral cancer if not treated. The standard treatment for leukoplakia is surgery, but this may not be feasible if the condition has spread over large areas of the mouth.

Q: Is treatment with Accutane successful?

A: It certainly shows promise. In one study, by researchers at the University of Texas M.D. Anderson Cancer Center, in Houston, Accutane was given in large doses to 70 people with leukoplakia. After three months, 24 of 53 of the people who responded well to this treatment were assigned to a lower, maintenance dose of the drug, while the rest were given beta-carotene. After nine months, the researchers found that only two of the people still taking the drug (8 percent) had worsening of their conditions. However, 16 (55 percent) of those taking beta-carotene experienced worsening.

Q: Sounds good—but are there any side effects associated with Accutane?

A: Yes. Dry eyes and mouth, headaches and depression are common in people taking large doses. That's why some researchers believe its use should be reserved for people who have severe leukoplakia or who've previously had oral cancer. Just what percentage of people are permanently cured of their leukoplakia by a course of several months of Accutane is unknown. Most people cannot take it in large doses for more than a year or so, but smaller, maintenance doses may be effective with fewer side effects, says researcher Scott M. Lippman, M.D.

We should mention here, before we move on, that large doses of beta-carotene have also been tried against oral leukoplakia, but beta-carotene doesn't seem to be as effective as Accutane at treating this condition. Still, some researchers are hopeful it will prove to be of some use, since it has no side effects.

Q: Are people supposed to get a certain amount of beta-carotene?

A: There is no RDA for beta-carotene. To meet the RDA for vitamin A, you'd need to get about six milligrams of beta-carotene a day.

Q: How much beta-carotene do people actually get each day?

A: Dietary surveys show that people get about 25 percent of the RDA for vitamin A from beta-carotene, which means they are getting about 1.5 milligrams of beta-carotene a day, a very small amount and nowhere near the 15 to 20 milligrams that reduced risks for cancer and other diseases in population studies.

Q: I've heard you can turn orange if you eat too many carrots or take too much beta-carotene as supplements. Is that true?

A: Yes, your skin can turn a yellow-orange color if you take more than 30 milligrams a day of beta-carotene. But this condition is harmless and goes away if you reduce the amount of beta-carotene you are consuming.

Q: Does anyone need greater-than-RDA amounts of vitamin A?

A: Some people may require more. People with absorption problems may need greater-than-average amounts of the vitamin; so may people who are recovering from extensive burns.

VITAMIN A AND BETA-CAROTENE QUICK-REFERENCE GUIDE

RDA
For men, 1,000 RE (5,000 I.U.); for women, 800 RE (4,000 I.U.)

SOURCES
Cod-liver oil, beef liver, oysters, butter, whole milk, egg yolks, and orange and green leafy vegetables, such as carrots, sweet potatoes, butternut squash, mangoes, apricots, spinach, turnip greens, bok choy, broccoli and romaine lettuce.

SIGNS OF DEFICIENCY
Night blindness; dry eyes and mouth; susceptibility to infection; swollen eyelids and sticky discharge from the eyes; coarse, rough skin.

POSSIBLE TOXICITY PROBLEMS
A single large dose of 250,000 to 300,000 I.U. or smaller amounts of 50,000 I.U. for long periods of time can cause symptoms of toxicity, such as bone and joint pain, hair loss, skin dryness, itching and flaking, weakness, headache and vision problems.

B-COMPLEX VITAMINS

The following vitamins—B$_6$, B$_{12}$, folic acid, niacin, thiamin, biotin, pantothenic acid and riboflavin—are part of the group known as B complex. These vitamins were originally grouped together because they were found in liver and brewer's yeast (sold in health-food stores and the same type of yeast that is used to brew beer and other kinds of alcohol) and thought to be just one vitamin. Eventually, however, they were found to vary in structure.

These vitamins do have many characteristics in common. All are water-soluble, and all are essential for the body's use of energy from foods and for normal tissue production.

Vitamin B$_6$

Q: **What is vitamin B$_6$?**

A: Vitamin B$_6$—a water-soluble B complex vitamin, as we just explained—comes in three chemically related forms. The most common form, pyridoxine, is used in vitamin supplements and food fortification.

Q: **In what foods is B$_6$ found?**

A: Many foods contain vitamin B$_6$. The richest sources are chicken, fish, liver, kidney, pork and eggs. Other good sources include brown rice, soybeans, oats, whole-wheat products, peanuts and walnuts.

Q: **Exactly what role does vitamin B$_6$ play in the body?**

A: Like most of the other B complex vitamins, B$_6$ works in the release of energy from food, a process called

metabolism. It helps convert the calories we take in as carbohydrates into usable energy, through complex chemical reactions that involve oxygen. Without a dietary source of B_6,
the carbohydrates we eat are incompletely metabolized,
allowing compounds to build up to toxic levels in the blood.
It's these toxic compounds that are thought to be an important cause of vitamin-deficiency symptoms.

Vitamin B_6 is required for the proper functioning of more
than 60 enzymes. It is converted in the liver, red blood cells
and other tissues into biochemicals necessary for metabolism.
It is also essential for the body's manufacture of **nucleic
acid**, the genetic building block for all cells.

Vitamin B_6 plays a role in cell multiplication, including the
red blood cells and cells of the immune system. Deficiencies
can cause anemia and lowered resistance to infection.

Q: Does B_6 play any role in cancer prevention?

A: It may, both through its effects on immune function
and proper cell replication. Low blood levels of B_6
have been found in people with breast cancer and Hodgkin's
disease (a cancer of the lymph glands). And animals deprived
of B_6 seem to be more vulnerable to virus-induced malig-
nant tumors.

Q: Does it have any other important functions?

A: Vitamin B_6 also influences the nervous system,
through its effect on minerals and neurotransmitters,
the messengers of the central nervous system. B_6 is necessary
for the body to convert tryptophan, a constituent of protein,
to serotonin, an important brain neurotransmitter with many
physiological functions. Concentrations of B_6 are up to 25 to
50 times higher in the brain than in the blood.

Q: What does vitamin B6 have to do with fighting infection?

A: Both animals and humans with B6 deficiencies have severely depressed immune responses, more so than with deficiencies of any other B vitamins. Many different aspects of the immune response are affected, including the number of infection-fighting white blood cells and their ability to identify a particular type of disease-causing invader and launch an attack. Many researchers believe that getting adequate amounts of vitamin B6 can improve immune response.

Researchers at the USDA Human Nutrition Research Center on Aging at Tufts University have shown that B6 supplements can boost immunity in older healthy people, reversing what was considered to be an age-related slowing down of the immune system that put them at risk for infection and, possibly, cancer.

Q: You said that B6 is essential for certain brain chemicals. Is vitamin B6 ever used to treat mental disorders?

A: Yes. Vitamin B6 has been used for a variety of mental symptoms, although its use is considered controversial. Researchers at Tufts University have reported that B vitamin supplements, including B6, improved symptoms of depression and mental performance in men ages 70 to 79 suffering from depression. In the study all the men were given an antidepressant medication, and half also took a supplement containing 10 milligrams each of B1, B2 and B6.

Q: A friend of mine takes vitamin B6 for carpal tunnel syndrome, a nerve problem she has in her hands from typing all day long. Is it proven to work for this?

A: Vitamin B6 does seem to help some cases of carpal tunnel syndrome, several studies show.

In this condition, a nerve that passes through the wrist, the median nerve, is compressed, causing a pins-and-needles sensation in the hands. A study by Allan L. Bernstein, M.D., chief neurologist at Kaiser-Permanente Medical Center, in Hayward, California, found reduced pain in people who took 150 mg. of B6 a day. Pain relief took 8 to 12 weeks to kick in. The dosage is maintained for a few months, then gradually reduced to a lower, maintenance dose.

Q: Isn't vitamin B6 sometimes also recommended to women who have premenstrual syndrome?

A: Yes. In two small studies, doses of 500 mg. of vitamin B6 did seem to provide some relief from symptoms of breast tenderness, headaches, fluid retention, irritability and nausea associated with premenstrual syndrome. We should add that this dosage borders on an amount that requires medical supervision.

Q: What else is vitamin B6 used for?

A: Daily doses seem to protect people from "Chinese restaurant syndrome"—headaches, flushing, rapid heartbeat and tightening around the temples and neck, which some people develop when they eat monosodium glutamate (MSG—an ingredient often used in Chinese food).

Vitamin B6 has been used for years to treat morning sickness, and a study by researchers at the University of Iowa College of Medicine found it really works. In pregnant women who took 25 mg. every 8 hours for 72 hours, vitamin B6 provided significant relief from severe nausea and vomiting, compared with a group taking placebos, or harmless blank pills. It appeared to have no effect on mild nausea, however.

Q: Anything else it's good for?

A: Some research also suggests that vitamin B6 deficiency may play a role in the development of some kinds of kidney stones, in raising risks for heart disease, in worsening some types of seizure disorders, and in the development of diabetes-associated cataracts. Some doctors use supplements of vitamin B6 and other B vitamins to help recovering alcoholics regain normal neurological and psychological function.

Q: Do people get enough B6?

A: Apparently a lot of people don't get enough. There is more evidence of low intakes of vitamin B6 than of any other vitamin, reports one nutrition textbook, *Nutrition and Physical Fitness* by George Briggs, Ph.D., and Doris Calloway, Ph.D., of the University of California at Berkeley. In a study by the USDA, the average intake for adult men in the United States was 1.87 mg. For women, it was 1.16 mg.

VITAMIN B6
QUICK-REFERENCE GUIDE

RDA
For men, 2 mg.; for women, 1.6 mg.

SOURCES
Vitamin B6 is widely distributed in foods. The richest sources are chicken, fish, liver, kidney, pork and eggs. Other good sources include brown rice, soybeans, oats, whole-wheat products, peanuts and walnuts.

SIGNS OF DEFICIENCY
Deficiency rarely occurs alone and is most commonly seen in people who are deficient in several B complex vitamins. Signs of deficiency include weakness; sleeplessness; nerve problems in hands and feet; inflamed lips, tongue and mouth; and reduced resistance to infection.

POSSIBLE TOXICITY PROBLEMS
Taken in large amounts for a long period of time, vitamin B6 can cause trouble walking and severe **sensory neuropathy**— loss of sensation in the feet and hands.
  Toxicity has been observed, although rarely, with doses of 100 to 200 mg. Most problems, however, observed in men or women have occurred at doses higher than 500 mg. a day.

Vitamin B_{12}

Q: What is vitamin B_{12}?

A: Vitamin B_{12} is a water-soluble vitamin and the last of the B vitamins to be discovered, in 1948. It has the most complex structure of any of the B vitamins, and is a bright red color. At its core is a molecule of cobalt, which explains its official name, cobalamin.

Q: In what foods is B_{12} found?

A: Liver and organ meats are the best sources. Muscle meats, fish, eggs, shellfish, milk and most dairy products, except butter, are good sources.

Q: What does B_{12} do in the body?

A: One of its important roles in the body is the manufacture of chemical compounds that support the growth and normal function of nerves and the spinal cord.

Q: What happens to the nervous system when B_{12} intake is low?

A: B_{12} deficiencies are linked to a deterioration in mental functioning, to neurological damage and to a number of psychological disturbances. B_{12} deficiency results in the deterioration of the fatty sheath covering nerves, a process called demyelination that often begins in the peripheral nerves and eventually moves to the spine.

Q: What are signs of deficiency?

A: In one study, 39 people with neurological symptoms related to B_{12} deficiency were treated with vitamin B_{12}. All showed improvement—sometimes dramatic improvement. Their symptoms included abnormal gait, memory loss, decreased reflexes, weakness, fatigue, disorientation, psychiatric disorders and impaired touch or pain sensation.

Other possible signs include symmetrical tingling or loss of sensation or weakness in hands or feet, diminished sensitivity to vibration and position sense, changes in personality or mood, and hallucinations.

Q: Is B_{12} important for anything else?

A: B_{12} is also essential for the normal functioning of all body cells, particularly those of the bone marrow (which produces red blood cells), the nervous system and the gastrointestinal tract.

And like B_6, vitamin B_{12} is needed for the body to make nucleic acids, the genetic material found in all cells.

Q: I've heard that this vitamin is supposed to give people an energy boost. Is that correct?

A: Years of clinical experience prove that people who have clear-cut vitamin B_{12} deficiencies perk up once they receive adequate amounts. Those people may have a potentially fatal form of anemia, called **pernicious anemia**, caused by the body's inability to produce normal red blood cells. This type of anemia produces abnormally large, elliptical blood cells. The blood also contains many fragments of blood cells and other microscopic signs of abnormalities.

And studies indicate that apparently more people than previously realized have subtle deficiencies, with no signs of anemia, and also gain more energy with increased intake of the nutrient.

Q: Any connection between vitamin B_{12} deficiencies and cancer?

A: There may well be links associated with its role in the manufacture of nucleic acid, which we mentioned earlier. In one study, supplementation with B_{12} and folic acid (another B vitamin involved in the manufacture of nucleic acid) helped to reverse potentially premalignant cell changes in the lungs of smokers.

Q: Do most people get enough B_{12}?

A: Yes. About the only people who don't get more than enough through their diets are vegans—strict vegetarians who don't eat meat, dairy products or eggs.

Q: Does that mean B_{12} deficiency is rare?

A: No. Deficiencies in vitamin B_{12} are not uncommon, and are due to problems absorbing the nutrient.

Q: Why can't some people absorb vitamin B_{12}?

A: They may have malabsorption problems due to certain diseases, such as celiac disease, or due to low amounts of stomach acid (a condition called *achlorhydria*), overgrowths of bacteria in the bowel, or previous stomach or intestinal surgery. Any of these conditions may make them unable to produce a protein called **intrinsic factor**, which escorts B_{12} through the bowel into the bloodstream.

Q: Then how do these people get their vitamin B12?

A: They may need regular B12 injections.

Q: Do many people have this problem and require injections?

A: Several recent studies found that many more older people than previously thought may have problems with vitamin B12 absorption, mostly due to inadequate production of stomach acid. In one study, almost 15 percent of people ages 65 to 99 had signs of low B12 levels. Other studies suggest that 5 to 10 percent of people age 65 or older have low levels of vitamin B12, often without signs of anemia.

Q: How can I be checked for a B12 deficiency?

A: Blood tests are used. Usually, a serum B12 test is done first. If that's low, doctors test to check for two other blood components associated with B12 deficiency: homocysteine and methylmalonic acid. Other tests are available to check for anemia and for the ability to absorb vitamin B12.

Several leading B12 researchers feel it's wise for everyone to begin periodic screening for B12 deficiency once they reach age 65. This is a test you'll probably have to request your doctor to perform, since most do not offer routine B12 testing and may not even recognize early signs of deficiency.

Q: Does vitamin B12 deficiency develop suddenly?

A: No. It often takes years to develop, with gradually worsening of symptoms related to nerves or mental functioning. Early detection can often prevent permanent nerve damage.

VITAMIN B12
QUICK-REFERENCE GUIDE

RDA
For men and women, 2 micrograms.

SOURCES
Found only in animal foods or foods fermented by bacteria.
The richest sources are liver and organ meats. Muscle meats,
fish, eggs, shellfish, milk and most dairy products, except
butter, are good sources.

SIGNS OF DEFICIENCY
Symmetrical tingling or loss of sensation or weakness in hands
or feet, diminished sensitivity to vibration and position sense,
trouble walking, memory loss, fatigue (often initially without
anemia), changes in personality or mood, and hallucinations.

POSSIBLE TOXICITY PROBLEMS
Vitamin B12 has no known toxicity. Dietary levels of at least
several hundred times the nutritional requirements are
considered safe.

Folic Acid

Q: What is folic acid?

A: Folic acid is a bright-yellow powder and one of the
water-soluble B complex vitamins. (Folic acid and
related compounds exhibiting the same properties as folic
acid are called folacin or folate.) The name comes from the
Latin word meaning "foliage" and was coined by researchers
who waded through four tons of spinach to come up with
the first pure samples of folic acid.

Q: So it's found in spinach? What about
other foods?

A: The richest sources of folic acid are liver, brewer's
yeast and dark green leafy vegetables, such as spinach
or kale. Good sources include dried beans, green vegetables

such as asparagus, lettuce and broccoli, fresh oranges and whole-wheat products.

Q: What exactly is brewer's yeast again?

A: The brewer's yeast sold in health-food stores is the same type of yeast that is used to brew beer and other kinds of alcohol. It is an excellent source of several nutrients, including thiamin, riboflavin, niacin, B_6, pantothenic acid, biotin and folic acid, as well as some essential minerals and trace minerals, especially chromium and selenium. It also contains an array of amino acids that may have an immune-enhancing effect. And it may contain other ingredients that enhance healing.

Q: Okay. Back to folic acid—what role does it play in the body?

A: Folic acid is essential for normal growth and re-production, for the prevention of blood disorders, and for important biochemical mechanisms within each cell. Folic acid is involved in the synthesis of nucleic acid, the genetic building blocks for all cells. Folic acid deficiencies have been associated with serious birth defects, with a certain type of anemia, and with increased risks for some types of cancer.

Q: How is folic acid associated with birth defects?

A: Several recent studies have found that women who are low in folic acid are at increased risk of having babies with neural-tube defects. These defects include fail-ure of the brain to develop and failure of the spinal column to close.

Other studies have shown that getting adequate folic acid reduces the risk of neural-tube defects, both in high-risk women—those who've previously had babies with such defects—and in women who are having a first child. Since these defects occur right around the time of conception, often before a woman knows she is pregnant, experts from the U.S. Public Health Service recommend that women of childbearing age have a daily intake of about 400 micrograms of folic acid. That's about twice what most get. Women who've previously had babies with neural-tube defects and who are planning to get pregnant should discuss the possibility of even higher doses with their doctors, experts say.

Some 2,500 babies are born each year with neural-tube defects, and it is estimated that another 1,500 are aborted during the second trimester, when neural-tube defects can be detected.

Q: How is folic acid associated with anemia? I thought anemia was caused by an iron deficiency.

A: Iron-deficiency anemia is only one of several types of anemia. Folic-acid deficiency causes a type of anemia called **macrocytic anemia**. In this form of anemia, the mature red blood cells are fewer in number, larger in size and contain less of the oxygen-carrying protein hemoglobin than normal. The young red blood cells in the bone marrow fail to mature in a person deficient in folic acid. Once adequate amounts of folic acid are given, the red blood cells promptly develop to maturity. Anemia caused by iron deficiency is not remedied by folic acid; on the other hand, anemia caused by a B_{12} deficiency does improve when folic acid is given.

Q: And what about cancer and folic acid?

A: In a study of men with potentially premalignant changes in the cells lining the lungs, supplements of 10 milligrams a day of folic acid, along with vitamin B_{12}, reduced the number of atypical cells. The researchers—

leaders in their field from the University of Alabama at
Birmingham—speculate that cigarette smoke might create a
folic-acid deficiency in the cells lining the lungs, making them
susceptible to damage from chemicals in cigarette smoke.

Low blood levels of folic acid have been associated with
an increased risk for **cervical dysplasia**—potentially premalignant changes in the cells lining the cervix. The researchers
speculate that low levels of folic acid make cervical cells
vulnerable to virus-induced damage. An earlier study by the
same researchers suggests that supplemental folic acid may
prevent dysplasia from becoming progressively abnormal or
even help it revert to normal.

Q: Are people likely to be low in this nutrient?

A: The answer depends on what you consider low.
Getting enough folic acid to meet the RDA used to be
considered a problem for many people. In 1989, however,
the RDA for folic acid was slashed in half—from 400 to 200
micrograms for men, and from 400 to 180 mcg. for women.
This is more in line with what people are actually consuming.
Some researchers consider the RDA is adequate; others think
it is too low, especially for women of childbearing age, since
adequate folic-acid intake at the time of conception is important for normal fetal development. Some preliminary
research also suggests that optimum amounts to prevent
chronic disease may be higher than RDA amounts.

Q: What are signs of deficiency?

A: Symptoms of folic-acid deficiency include fatigue,
loss of appetite, anemia, inflamed tongue (which
often feels like a burning sensation), gastrointestinal
problems and diarrhea.

**FOLIC ACID
QUICK-REFERENCE GUIDE**

RDA
For men, 200 mcg., for women, 180 mcg.

SOURCES
The richest sources are liver, brewer's yeast and dark green leafy vegetables. Good sources include dried beans, green vegetables such as asparagus, lettuce and broccoli, fresh oranges and whole-wheat products.

SIGNS OF DEFICIENCY
Fatigue, loss of appetite, anemia, inflamed tongue, gastro-intestinal problems and diarrhea.

POSSIBLE TOXICITY PROBLEMS
Toxicity is considered rare, and not all studies have produced signs of toxicity, even at very high doses. In one study, doses of 15 grams a day caused gastrointestinal problems and sleep disturbances. Doses of 8 grams or more may cause neuro-logical injury when given to people with undiagnosed pernicious anemia.

Folic acid can interfere with the effectiveness of antiseizure drugs. People taking drugs that interfere with the body's ability to use folic acid, used for cancer, arthritis or other conditions, should take folic acid only with their doctor's approval.

Niacin

Q: What is niacin?

A: Niacin is one of the B vitamins, sometimes also known as B₃. It is a white powder, soluble in water and more resistant to destruction than any of the other B complex vitamins. Niacin includes both **nicotinic acid** and **nicotinamide**, also sometimes called **niacinamide**. Both forms of niacin perform basically the same functions, but nicotinic acid has the additional talent of lowering blood cholesterol levels. It also produces side effects not found with nicotinamide.

Q: In what foods is niacin found?

A: The richest sources are brewer's yeast, wheat bran and peanuts. Good sources include chicken, tuna, turkey, beef and whole-grain wheat products. Fruits, vegetables and dairy products all contain a bit of niacin.

Q: What role does niacin perform in the body?

A: Like the other B vitamins, niacin is crucial for the body's manufacture of enzymes that provide the body with energy and the building blocks for cell reproduction and repair. It is known to be involved in more than 200 enzymatic reactions in the body involving the metabolism of carbohydrates, fats and proteins. Further, niacin has been identified as part of the chromium-containing **glucose tolerance factor** found in brewer's yeast, which enhances the body's response to **insulin**. (Insulin is a hormone that helps to transport **glucose**—blood sugar—into cells and to store it in the liver and muscles.)

Niacin is carried in the blood and is found in all tissues, but most abundantly in the liver, kidney, heart, brain and muscles. A lack of niacin can cause cell damage anywhere in the body.

Q: What did you say earlier about niacin and cholesterol?

A: Large doses of about two grams a day of one form of niacin, nicotinic acid, are sometimes used to help lower blood cholesterol and **triglyceride** levels, both of which are known to be involved in the development of coronary-artery disease.

Research has found that nicotinic acid markedly lowers harmful **LDL** (low-density lipoproteins) in the blood while raising levels of heart-healthy **HDL** (high-density lipoproteins). One major study also found that the use of nicotinic acid reduced the recurrence of heart attacks in men with heart disease by almost 30 percent. The bad news, unfortunately, is that large doses of nicotinic acid produce undesirable side effects.

Q: **Hold on there—what kinds of side effects are you talking about?**

A: Doses in the hundreds of milligrams can cause flushing of the skin and intense itching. Doses in the thousands of milligrams can cause liver damage, which may first appear as **jaundice**, a liver disorder that causes a yellowing of the eyes and skin. Some doctors consider timed-release nicotinic acid more likely to cause liver problems than regular nicotinic acid.

Q: **What else is niacin used for?**

A: Niacin has been used successfully, along with the amino acid tryptophan, in the treatment of depression. It apparently enhances the effect of tryptophan in maintaining adequate blood levels of an important brain neurotransmitter, serotonin.

Nicotinic acid has also been used as a therapy to dilate blood vessels and, thus, increase blood flow to certain areas of the body, to stimulate tooth eruption, to increase the flow of gastric juices and to increase intestinal motility—the action of the intestines to move food along.

Q: **Does niacin play any role in cancer protection?**

A: Preliminary research shows that it apparently plays a prime role in cancer prevention. A form of niacin is involved in the body's production of a substance that repairs the kind of genetic damage that may occur with exposure to viruses or harmful drugs, say scientists at the Texas College of Osteopathic Medicine, in Fort Worth, Texas. If the body lacks niacin, however, cell damage goes unrepaired and cancer may develop. Research is currently under way to determine in humans how different niacin intakes affect the body's ability to repair genetic damage to cells.

Q: What else can niacin do?

A: The same study that found that people taking large amounts of niacin had reduced risk for a second heart attack also found that people taking large amounts of niacin had significantly lower death rates in *every* cause-of-death category analyzed: coronary disease, other cardiovascular diseases, cancer and all other causes. Niacin has been prescribed to reduce symptoms during alcohol or drug withdrawal, to treat schizophrenia and some other mental disorders, to relieve migraine headaches, and to relieve symptoms of diabetes and arthritis. But there are few studies to prove that it helps any of these conditions.

Q: How much niacin do people get in their diets?

A: The average American diet provides about 20 mg. a day, which is close to the RDA. So niacin isn't considered a problem nutrient.

Q: What are signs of deficiency?

A: The classic niacin deficiency disease, pellagra, means "rough skin" in Italian. Symptoms of this potentially fatal disease, once common in the American South in people surviving mostly on corn, include what nutrition students call "the 3-Ds"—dermatitis, diarrhea and dementia. More specific symptoms include irritability, anxiety and depression, sore mouth and tongue, inflamed membranes in the intestinal tract (with bloody diarrhea in the later stages), and a reddish skin rash, especially on the face, hands and feet when they are exposed to sunlight, which later makes the skin rough and dark.

The same signs of niacin deficiency just noted are thought to also include problems with tryptophan deficiency and metabolism and with vitamin B_6. Tryptophan is an amino acid that can be converted to niacin, and vitamin B_6 is necessary for the conversion. Large amounts of tryptophan in the diet can overcome a niacin-poor diet.

NIACIN
QUICK-REFERENCE GUIDE

RDA
For men, 19 mg.; for women, 15 mg.

SOURCES
Richest sources are brewer's yeast, wheat bran and peanuts. Good sources include chicken, tuna, turkey, beef and whole-grain wheat products. Fruits, vegetables and dairy products all contain a bit of niacin.

SIGNS OF DEFICIENCY
Irritability, anxiety, depression, sore mouth and tongue, inflamed membranes in the intestinal tract (with bloody diarrhea in the later stages), and a reddish skin rash, especially on the face, hands and feet when they are exposed to sunlight, which later makes the skin rough and dark.

POSSIBLE TOXICITY PROBLEMS
Doses of several hundred milligrams of nicotinic acid can cause flushing of the skin and intense itching. Doses of 1,500 to 3,000 milligrams can cause jaundice and have the potential to cause liver damage. About one-third of people on high-dose therapy show abnormal results in one or more tests of liver function. In most cases, liver function returns to normal once nicotinic acid is stopped. Severe heartburn, nausea and vomiting may also occur at high doses.

Thiamin

Q: **What is thiamin?**

A: Thiamin is a B complex vitamin. It was the first to be obtained in a pure form, which is why it is also sometimes called vitamin B_1. Thiamin deficiency causes the disease traditionally known as beriberi, which is characterized by numbness and tingling in toes and feet, stiffness of the ankles, cramping pains in the legs, difficulty walking, and finally paralysis of the legs with wasting of leg muscles.

Q: **I've seen the word spelled with an "e" on the end. Is thiamine the same nutrient as thiamin?**

A: That's an old spelling still sometimes used by the Food and Drug Administration and some other authorities.

Q: **What foods are good sources of thiamin?**

A: Not many foods are great sources. Those that are include brewer's yeast, organ meats, whole grains, pork and beans. Foods with moderate amounts of thiamin include meat, fish and poultry, eggs, nuts, milk and dairy products, vegetables and thiamin-enriched flours and cereals. Oatmeal and dried beans are a good, economical source of thiamin.

Q: **What role does thiamin play in the body?**

A: Like most of the other B complex vitamins, thiamin works in the release of energy from food. It helps our bodies convert the calories we take in as carbohydrates into usable energy, through complex chemical reactions that involve oxygen. Without a dietary source of thiamin, the carbohydrates we eat are incompletely metabolized, allowing compounds to build up to toxic levels in the blood. It's these toxic compounds that are thought to be an important cause of deficiency symptoms, such as the nerve problems and muscle wasting seen in beriberi.

Thiamin is essential for nearly every cellular reaction in the body—for normal development, growth, reproduction, maximum physical fitness and good health. It's needed for normal skin and hair, brain and nerve function, blood production and normal defense against infections and disease.

Q: Is thiamin used to treat any diseases?

A: Thiamin has been used to help treat some of the symptoms associated with alcohol abuse, such as mental confusion, visual disturbances and staggering gait. As we mentioned before, alcoholics are usually deficient in this vitamin.

Thiamin deficiency can contribute to heart disease. For people with low thiamin levels, getting adequate amounts may help to correct symptoms of disturbed heart rhythm, shortness of breath, swelling of the feet and legs, low blood pressure and chest pain.

Q: Any other problems thiamin helps?

A: Thiamin deficiency can cause a variety of nerve problems, and thiamin has been used to treat deficiency-related nerve problems, such as generalized muscle weakness and paralysis, especially of the eye muscles. However, claims that thiamin can help neurological disorders unrelated to deficiency, such as multiple sclerosis, Bell's palsy and myasthenia gravis, have not been substantiated.

An unusual form of anemia also responds to large doses of thiamin. And thiamin-deficient diabetic people who are restored to normal intake usually see an improvement in blood-sugar metabolism.

Q: Are there any mental symptoms of thiamin deficiency, as there are with other B complex vitamins?

A: Yes. Thiamin has been called "the morale vitamin" because one of the earliest signs of its lack is reduced stamina. Studies of people who voluntarily followed a diet moderately low in thiamin found that they developed symptoms in as few as 10 days. They became depressed and irritable, and lacked the ability to concentrate on and take an interest in their work. Additional symptoms appeared in 3 to 10 weeks, and included fatigue, lack of appetite, weight loss, constipation, muscle cramps and various pains. The subjects recovered promptly when given larger amounts of thiamin.

Q: Do most people get enough thiamin from their diets?

A: Studies show that most Americans get enough thiamin to prevent full-blown beriberi, which is characterized by numbness and tingling in toes and feet, stiffness of ankles, cramping pains in the legs and other symptoms. But many diets provide less than optimal amounts, especially during times of physical stress, such as pregnancy, illness or surgery. Alcoholism also contributes to thiamin deficiencies by depleting body stores of the nutrient. The need for thiamin also increases along with the number of calories a day you burn.

Q: Who is likely to be deficient?

A: In the United States, chronic alcoholics often show nervous-system symptoms associated with a thiamin deficiency, such as numbness and tingling in the toes and feet. That's because their diets often lack this nutrient and their high intake of calories in the form of alcohol increases their need for thiamin. Alcohol also reduces thiamin absorption from the intestine, a problem so prevalent among alcoholics that public-health officials in at least one country, Australia, have considered fortifying beer with thiamin.

Others at risk of getting too little thiamin include those on weight-loss diets, heavy coffee or tea drinkers, very old people, and people taking drugs such as furosemide (Lasix, a diuretic), digoxin and antacids.

Q: **Didn't you say earlier that physical stress and exercise potentially put a person a risk for thiamin deficiency?**

A: Yes. People who exercise a lot and eat lots of carbohydrates need more thiamin than those who are muscularly inactive. For that reason, the RDA for thiamin is usually stated in terms of the caloric intake—so much for every 1,000 calories. However, no matter how few calories a person is eating, the minimum amount remains at just over one milligram a day.

THIAMIN
QUICK-REFERENCE GUIDE

RDA
For men, 1.5 mg.; for women, 1.1 mg.

SOURCES
Few foods are rich sources of thiamin. Those that are include brewer's yeast, organ meats, whole grains, pork and beans. Foods with moderate amounts of thiamin include thiamin-enriched flours and cereals, meat, fish and poultry, eggs, nuts, milk and dairy products, and vegetables. Oatmeal and dried beans are a good, economical source of thiamin.

SIGNS OF DEFICIENCY
Numbness or tingling in toes and feet, stiffness, cramping pains in the legs, difficulty in walking, digestive problems, lack of appetite, fatigue, depression, irritability.

POSSIBLE TOXICITY PROBLEMS
Long-term toxicity can produce symptoms of **hyperthyroidism**: headache, irritability, trembling, rapid pulse and insomnia. With injected thiamin, reactions of itching, weakness, pain, sweating, nausea, tingling and faintness have occurred at varying amounts. Five milligrams daily is the lowest oral dose known to cause side effects, but most people apparently tolerate much higher amounts with no ill effects. Reports of side effects are rare.

Biotin

Q: What is biotin?

A: Biotin is a water-soluble B complex vitamin that is produced in our intestines as well as being obtained from foods.

Q: What role does biotin play in the body?

A: Like the other B vitamins, biotin is essential for the body's metabolism of carbohydrates and fats, and for making protein. It plays a crucial part in the production of nucleic acid, the substance from which a cell's genetic material is formed.

Q: Is biotin used to treat any medical conditions?

A: Horses and pigs with severe splitting hooves are helped with supplemental doses of biotin, and a study by Swiss researchers shows that this vitamin also improves in humans the condition of splitting, frail, soft or thin fingernails, caused by a breakdown of the intercellular cement between the hard layers of nail tissue.

Biotin may also help some skin disorders, such as seborrheic dermatitis, an oily, scaly condition of the scalp, face, chest, back, underarms and groin.

Large doses of biotin are also used to treat a rare and potentially fatal genetic inability to utilize biotin in the body.

Q: Don't I recall seeing a shampoo or two that contained biotin?

A: Yes. Some shampoos do contain this vitamin, although most experts agree it's unlikely to do any good in this form.

On the positive side, though, oral supplementation with biotin has been successful in the management of "uncombable hair syndrome," a disorder in children that causes hair to stick up in all directions.

Q: So biotin deficiency is a problem for hair?

A: Yes. Biotin deficiency does cause hair loss, and in people who are low in biotin, increased amounts can restore hair. But most people with hair loss are not biotin deficient, and no amount of biotin is going to restore their hair.

Q: Is biotin deficiency common?

A: No, it's considered to be fairly uncommon. Studies show that most people get about 100 to 200 micrograms of biotin a day.

BIOTIN
QUICK-REFERENCE GUIDE

RDA
No RDA, but an Estimated Safe and Adequate Daily Dietary Intake of 30 to 100 mcg. for men and women.

SOURCES
Liver, kidney, brewer's yeast, egg yolks, whole grains, breads, fish, nuts, beans, meat and dairy products.

SIGNS OF DEFICIENCY
In adults, loss of hair; a scaly red rash around the nose, mouth and other body orifices; intense depression; hallucinations; sleeplessness and muscle pain. In infants, signs also include profound development delay and a lack of muscle tone.

POSSIBLE TOXICITY PROBLEMS
No evidence of toxicity.

Pantothenic Acid

Q: What is pantothenic acid?

A: It's also a water-soluble B complex vitamin. The word pantothenic is derived from the Greek, meaning "from everywhere." That name was given because this vitamin is present in all foods, although not always in substantial amounts.

Q: What role does pantothenic acid play in the body?

A: Pantothenic acid is involved in proper skin growth and nerve function, and in maintaining the health of the **adrenal glands**, which may become enlarged, reddened and prone to hemorrhage with pantothenic-acid deficiency. Pantothenic acid is known to be involved in the production of cortisone and two other related hormones produced by the adrenal glands. These hormones play an important role in metabolism and in the body's reaction to stress, including inflammation.

Claims that pantothenic acid prevents or alleviates arthritis have been examined in several studies. One double-blind study found "highly significant effects for oral calcium pantothenate [a form of pantothenic acid] in reducing the duration of morning stiffness, degree of disability and severity of pain" in patients suffering from rheumatoid arthritis, a form characterized by inflammation in the joints and elsewhere in the body.

Q: Does it do anything else?

A: Yes. Like other B vitamins, pantothenic acid plays a vital role in energy metabolism. It's essential for the breakdown and release of energy from carbohydrates, fats and proteins.

Studies examining the claims that pantothenic acid boosts energy and athletic ability have been mixed, however. In one study, well-trained distance runners who were given two grams of pantothenic acid a day for two weeks outperformed other, equally well-trained runners who received placebos. Those who got the pantothenic acid needed less oxygen to perform equivalent work and had significantly less buildup of the biochemicals produced during exercise that cause muscle soreness.

PANTOTHENIC ACID
QUICK-REFERENCE GUIDE

RDA
There is currently no RDA for pantothenic acid, but an Estimated Safe and Adequate Daily Dietary Intake of 4–7 mg. is recommended for men and women.

SOURCES
Foods especially rich in pantothenic acid include brewer's yeast, liver, eggs, wheat germ and bran, peanuts and peas. Good sources include meat, milk, poultry, whole grains, broccoli, mushrooms and sweet potatoes. Most vegetables and fruits contain small amounts.

SIGNS OF DEFICIENCY
Fatigue, headache, sleep disturbances, personality changes, nausea, abdominal distress, numbness and tingling of the hands and feet, burning sensations in the feet, muscle cramps, impaired coordination and immune problems.

POSSIBLE TOXICITY PROBLEMS
Most experts consider the risk of toxicity to be extremely low. In humans, dosages considered very large—10 to 20 grams a day—have not produced reactions more severe than mild diarrhea and fluid retention.

Riboflavin

Q: What is riboflavin?

A: Riboflavin is one of the B complex vitamins. It is a yellow-orange water-soluble compound, and, since it was second to be discovered, is sometimes also called vitamin B_2.

Q: What role does riboflavin play in the body?

A: Like other B complex vitamins, riboflavin is needed for the conversion of food to energy. It is carried through the blood to all cells in the body, where it is used to make enzymes important for energy metabolism. Riboflavin-containing compounds are essential for the metabolism of carbohydrates, amino acids and fats.

These compounds are also crucial for the proper development and maintenance of nerves and blood cells, for iron metabolism, for adrenal gland function, for the formation of connective tissues, and for proper immune function. So it's easy to see why a riboflavin deficiency can have an impact on the entire body.

Q: Has a deficiency been linked with any particular illness?

A: In studies, riboflavin deficiency has been associated with an increase in throat cancers and with the development of cataracts, a clouding of the lenses of the eyes that can lead to blindness.

Deficiency may also impair brain function. In one study, healthy people older than age 60 who got the RDA of riboflavin performed better on tests to assess memory than those getting less then the RDA of riboflavin.

RIBOFLAVIN
QUICK-REFERENCE GUIDE

RDA
For men, 1.7 mg.; for women, 1.3 mg.

SOURCES
Riboflavin is found in many different foods. The richest sources include organ meats such as liver, kidney and heart. Dark green leafy vegetables are also a good source. However, most Americans get their riboflavin from meats and dairy products, along with riboflavin-enriched white flour and cereals.

SIGNS OF DEFICIENCY
Skin problems, including a greasy, scaly condition on the face, are common signs of a severe deficiency. Red, swollen, cracked lips, especially at the corners on the mouth, and a sore, red tongue may also occur, along with loss of appetite, weakness, fatigue, depression and anemia, dimness of vision and burning of the eyes. Decreased sensitivity to touch, temperature, vibration and position may occur in the hands and feet.

POSSIBLE TOXICITY PROBLEMS
Risk of toxicity is very low. Probably because high doses are not well absorbed, high oral doses of riboflavin are essentially nontoxic.

VITAMIN C

Q: What is vitamin C?

A: Vitamin C, or **ascorbic acid**, is a white powder that dissolves easily in water. It's perhaps best known for its alleged ability to prevent colds, which we discuss in a bit, and it also plays a major role in many body functions. Vitamin C is the body's most powerful water-soluble antioxidant. It shields cells in the body from oxidative damage, a process we explain in detail later.

Q: In what foods is vitamin C found?

A: Think *C* for citrus, for starters. Oranges and grape-fruits are good sources. Other fruits rich in vitamin C include strawberries, kiwifruit, black currants, guava and papaya. Vegetables also offer a healthy share. Among the best bets for vitamin C are red bell peppers, broccoli and brussels sprouts. If you follow the suggestion of the National Academy of Sciences to eat at least five servings of fruits and vegetables a day, you'll get at least 120 milligrams of vitamin C—twice the RDA of 60 milligrams.

Q: What function does vitamin C play in the body?

A: Vitamin C has a variety of roles, all indispensable to good health. It is needed for the body to make connective tissue, or **collagen**, which is found throughout the body and helps maintain the structure of tissues, including skin, muscles, gums, blood vessels and bone. In the classic deficiency disease, scurvy, which has been recognized for more than 35 centuries, a lack of vitamin C leads to the breaking open of small blood vessels, the reddening and bleeding of skin and gums, loose teeth, general weakness and death.

Like vitamin E and beta-carotene, vitamin C also acts as an antioxidant. That means it helps to neutralize potentially harmful reactions in the body—reactions that can lead to cell damage associated with cancer, heart disease and an array of other health problems.

Q: But what does this mean in terms of health or disease?

A: Lots of claims have been made regarding vitamin C, and studies are showing that, at least in some cases, the claims are valid. Vitamin C has been found to help prevent—not cure—cancer, to boost immunity against colds and other infections, to combat heart disease and to speed wound healing and help prevent bedsores. It also appears to help overcome some types of male infertility and, in smokers, may even help to prevent sperm abnormalities that can lead to birth defects. It seems to counteract asthma, protect lungs against smoking and various pollutants, reduce some kinds of allergic response, and help prevent cataracts.

Q: Whew! Let's take these one at a time. How is vitamin C thought to help prevent cancer?

A: Studies done in the last decade or so show that vitamin C offers strong protection from cancer. Of 46 population studies that looked at vitamin C intake, 33 found a significantly reduced risk for cancer in people with the highest intake.

"In many of these studies, people getting the most vitamin C had about half as much risk for cancer as people with the lowest intake," says Gladys Block, Ph.D., a professor of nutrition at the University of California School of Public Health. High amounts of vitamin C were generally 150 mg. or more a day; low amounts, 60 mg. or less. That difference was equivalent to about four ounces of orange juice.

The protective effect seems to be strongest for cancers of the esophagus, larynx, mouth and pancreas. The nutrient also seems to provide some protection against cancers of the stomach, rectum, breast, cervix and perhaps even the lungs, Dr. Block says.

Q: What's the protective mechanism at work here?

A: Researchers say that vitamin C may shield against cancer by (1) helping protect a cell's genetic material from damage that can lead to cancerous changes; (2) by neutralizing chemical compounds such as nitrosamines— preservatives (often found in cold cuts and bacon) that increase your odds for gastrointestinal cancer; and (3) by beefing up your immune system's ability to track down and destroy precancerous cells.

Q: And what's the story on colds? Does vitamin C really knock them out?

A: Some people swear it works, and in fact, an analysis of a dozen studies of vitamin C's effect on colds shows a 37 percent average reduction in the duration of colds treated with vitamin C. In several studies, the number of days sick was cut from about a week to 5 days. Most of the studies also report a reduction in the severity of symptoms, such as sneezing, coughing and sniffling.

Q: How does vitamin C work against colds?

A: Vitamin C lowers blood levels of histamine, a bio-chemical (released by immune cells) that can trigger tissue inflammation and runny noses. It may also shield both immune cells and surrounding tissue from the oxidative reactions that occur when immune cells fight bacteria.

Q: What about heart disease? How's vitamin C supposed to prevent that?

A: Vitamin C helps prevent an apparent first step in the development of heart disease—the **oxidation** of artery-clogging LDL cholesterol. Oxidation is a chemical process in which a molecule combines with oxygen and loses electrons. Once LDL cholesterol is oxidized, it quickly turns into hard, artery-narrowing deposits.

In a study by researchers at the UCLA School of Public Health, high vitamin C intake was more strongly associated with reduced risk of heart disease than either low cholesterol levels or low-fat diet. The study found that men with the highest vitamin C intake—an average of 140 milligrams a day of vitamin C from foods and pills—had a death rate 42 percent lower than predicted. However, most researchers think current evidence of heart protection is stronger for vitamin E and beta-carotene than for vitamin C.

Q: How is vitamin C supposed to prevent bedsores?

A: It's well documented that vitamin C deficiencies lead to slower wound healing. And in a recent study by English researchers of people confined to bed because of hip fractures, low levels of vitamin C increased risk of developing bedsores.

Q: And male infertility problems? What is vitamin C supposed to do for those?

A: Researchers have found that a common form of male infertility, caused by sperm cells clumping together, can be reversed with supplementation of about one gram daily of vitamin C. Researchers at the University of California at Berkeley have also found that low intakes of vitamin C increase genetic damage in sperm cells, which could lead to birth defects. When test subjects increased their intakes of vitamin C to 60 mg. or even higher, genetic damage dropped.

Q: How is vitamin C supposed to protect against asthma or air pollution?

A: Vitamin C acts as an antioxidant in the lungs and, so, may help protect lungs from the damaging effects of cigarette smoke and air pollutants. In studies, exposure to cigarette smoke or air pollutants such as ozone depleted vitamin C in the lungs.

Because of its antihistamine and anti-inflammatory actions, vitamin C may also make lungs less reactive to spasm-causing irritants and, so, help reduce asthma and allergy attacks. One study showed that a 500 mg. dose of vitamin C taken an hour and a half before vigorous exercise lessened bronchial spasms in some people with asthma.

Q: And what about cataracts? Can vitamin C prevent them?

A: Cataracts occur when proteins in the eye's lens oxidize, turning an opaque, milky white.

In animal studies, vitamin C has been found to protect eye lenses against ultraviolet damage, reducing the incidence of cataracts. And in a recent study of 77 men and women with cataracts and 35 without, an important difference seemed to be how much fresh yellow, green and red fruits and vegetables they ate. Eating fewer than 3 ½ servings a day increased their risk of cataracts nearly sixfold.

Q: What does vitamin C have to do with the eye?

A: Vitamin C is highly concentrated in the lens of the eye, which may contain 60 times the amount of vitamin C found in the blood, says Allen Taylor, Ph.D., associate professor of biochemistry and nutrition at Tufts University and director of the laboratory for nutrition and vision research at the USDA Human Nutrition Research Center on Aging. It's possible that vitamin C helps protect the clear lens tissue from oxidative damage resulting from exposure to sunlight. Vitamin C may also protect enzymes within the lens that remove oxidation-damaged proteins, Dr. Taylor says, helping the eye heal itself.

Q: How much vitamin C are people supposed to get?

A: The RDA for vitamin C is 60 mg. a day. A recommendation of 100 milligrams a day for smokers, the first RDA to establish smokers as a special-needs group, was established in 1989, based on research showing that cigarette smoking depletes vitamin C in the body. And other studies have shown that amounts above the RDA are necessary to provide optimum vitamin C protection against the cell damage caused by free radicals.

Q: I know you mentioned this already but run it by me again. What are free radicals and how do they damage cells?

A: Free radicals are unbalanced molecular particles that are generated during reactions that involve oxygen and can damage cells by stealing away electrons. Free radicals have the potential to set off chain reactions of damage, but these reactions can be stopped if antioxidants such as vitamins C and E are present. Such vitamins offer up electrons to free radicals without becoming unbalanced themselves.

Q: Okay—back to vitamin C. Do people get enough of it?

A: Based on U.S. Department of Agriculture surveys, it is estimated that women in the United States get an average of 77 mg. of vitamin C a day, the amount found in 4 to 5 ounces of orange juice. The average intake for men is 109 mg. Researchers point out that it's hard to calculate exactly how much people are actually getting, however, since vitamin C is easily lost during storage and cooking.

VITAMIN C
QUICK-REFERENCE GUIDE

RDA
For men and women, 60 mg. daily. For smokers, 100 mg.

SOURCES
Very good sources are citrus fruits, red bell peppers, black currants and guava. Good sources include strawberries, kiwifruit, broccoli, brussels sprouts and papaya.

SIGNS OF DEFICIENCY
Easy bruising (capillary fragility), bleeding gums, muscular weakness, swollen or painful joints, nosebleeds, frequent infections, slow healing of wounds.

POSSIBLE TOXICITY PROBLEMS
Considered quite safe, even in large amounts, since the body simply excretes any vitamin C it can't use. Doses as low as 500 mg. can cause diarrhea in some people, but many people can take much larger doses with no problems. In one study, two of nine people taking 2,000 mg. of vitamin C a day suffered dry nose and nosebleeds.

People prone to gout or kidney stones or people with kidney diseases should take large amounts only with medical supervision. Scurvy has been reported in one case where a man taking 1,000 mg. a day of vitamin C abruptly stopped taking this supplement. Slowly reducing the dosage can prevent this.

VITAMIN D

Q:

What is vitamin D?

A:

Like vitamins A, E and K, vitamin D is a fat-soluble vitamin. In its pure form, it is a white crystal. As a supplement, however, it is usually found as a light yellow oil. It may be derived from cod-liver oil, which has 425 I.U. of vitamin D per teaspoon.

Vitamin D is unique from other vitamins in two ways: First, it can be synthesized in the skin from sunlight, which is why it is sometimes called the sunshine vitamin. Given enough exposure to sunlight, you need consume no vitamin D at all in the foods you eat. Second, vitamin D is the only

vitamin whose biologically active form is a hormone—
calcitriol. Vitamin D is converted into this hormone in the
kidneys before it performs its role in the body.

Q: What is the RDA of vitamin D?

A: It's 400 I.U. for men and for women ages 11 to 24;
and it's 200 I.U. for women age 25 or older.

Q: What are the best sources of vitamin D?

A: Vitamin D is not very abundant in the food chain. It
is mainly found in fatty fish, such as mackerel, tuna
and salmon, and in liver, eggs yolks and, to some extent,
milk fat.

Most milk sold in the United States is fortified with
vitamin D. One quart of whole, low-fat or skim milk offers
400 I.U. of vitamin D—100 percent of the RDA. Fortified
milk and infant formulas are the major dietary sources of
vitamin D in the United States.

Q: What does vitamin D do?

A: Vitamin D's most important role is the regulation of
two minerals, calcium and phosphorus. Both minerals
are important for normal growth and development, especially
the mineralization (hardening) of bone.

Vitamin D stimulates the absorption of calcium from the
gut. Without it, calcium cannot be absorbed. It also helps
harden bones and stimulates the kidneys to reabsorb some
calcium, thus saving the body from excreting calcium.

Q: What happens to bones if you're not getting enough vitamin D?

A: If you become vitamin D-deficient, your body increases production of a hormone that removes calcium from your bones.

In children, the classic vitamin D-deficiency disease is rickets, a condition characterized by bones so soft that they develop curves. Children with rickets are bowlegged or knock-kneed. The adult equivalent of rickets, a condition called **osteomalacia**, is also characterized by soft bones. Symptoms include bone pain and tenderness, and muscle weakness.

Q: Does low vitamin D intake play a role in the development of osteoporosis?

A: Apparently. "Even in the face of estrogen deficiency, which is generally considered to be the precipitating cause of osteoporosis, getting adequate vitamin D is important for preventing the bone loss associated with osteoporosis," says Michael Holick, M.D., Ph.D., director of the vitamin D laboratory at the Boston University School of Medicine.

In fact, a study by researchers at the USDA Human Nutrition Research Center on Aging at Tufts University, in Boston, found that postmenopausal women who took 400 I.U. of vitamin D (twice their RDA) daily reduced wintertime bone loss and improved bone density when compared with women who got approximately 100 I.U. of vitamin D a day. Both groups of women also took a supplement of calcium every day. It wasn't until the second winter, however, that the bone loss was greater in the placebo group than in the vitamin D-supplemented group.

Q: Is vitamin D beneficial in other ways in the body?

A: Preliminary research suggests that vitamin D, like vitamin A, may play a role in normal cell growth and maturation, which means it might help prevent cancer. It also seems to be involved in the regulation of the immune system, which could be important in the prevention and treatment of infectious diseases.

Q: **Does vitamin D have anything to do with cancer?**

A: Researchers don't know for sure. Colorectal and breast-cancer rates are highest, however, in areas where people are exposed to the least amount of natural sunlight. That correlation is found worldwide, except in Japan, where, researchers point out, people tend to eat lots of vitamin D-rich fatty fish, such as mackerel and salmon.

In laboratory experiments, the hormone form of vitamin D, calcitriol, does have anticancer properties. It has recently been found to inhibit the growth of human colon-cancer and skin-cancer cells in test-tube experiments. Calcitriol may also play a role in the treatment of retinoblastoma, the most common eye tumor of childhood. It has been found to inhibit the growth of this kind of tumor in mice.

Q: **And what about immune function?**

A: So far there's no solid proof that vitamin D plays a role in building immunity. But some researchers speculate that one reason sunlight seems to be helpful to people with conditions like tuberculosis is that it stimulates the body's production of vitamin D. Two test-tube studies have recently shown that the hormone form of vitamin D, calcitriol, stimulates the production of macrophages, immune cells that gobble up bacteria. However, there's little research on vitamin D's possible role in immune function in humans, according to Dr. Holick.

Q: How much vitamin D do most people get?

A: Studies show that most people don't reach the RDA of vitamin D from the foods they eat. Data from the U.S. Department of Agriculture show that most men get about 80 I.U. and most women about 60 I.U. of vitamin D from foods. In one study, men and women ages 60 to 93 years averaged about 50 I.U. of a day of vitamin D from foods.

Q: That seems low. Does exposure to the sun make up for the low intake from foods?

A: Dr. Holick tells us that "it is well documented that most people, in spring, summer and fall, get enough sunlight to make up for shortcomings in their diet. Even minimal exposure due to daily activities—such as going in and out of offices or playing tennis—is more than adequate." During winter months, however, blood levels of vitamin D tend to drop. And not everyone gets even the minimal amount of sunlight needed.

Q: Who's at risk for a vitamin D deficiency?

A: People in nursing homes or who simply don't go out much won't get the sunlight they need to maintain adequate vitamin D levels, Dr. Holick says. "We did a nursing-home study and found that upwards of 60 percent of people had low blood levels, even at the end of the summer."

Older people also do not manufacture vitamin D in their bodies as well as younger people. And they may consume low amounts of vitamin D-containing foods and take drugs that interfere with the absorption or metabolism of vitamin D. Such drugs include cholestyramine (used to control cholesterol and certain cases of diarrhea), mineral oil and certain anti-convulsants.

Q: Anyone else at risk?

A: Other people who may be at risk include alcoholics, people who don't drink milk or who don't get much sunlight, people with absorption problems, and those who live in areas where they receive little sunlight. African-Americans may be at higher risk, too, Dr. Holick says. "Their skin acts as a natural sunscreen, so they manufacture less vitamin D than light-skinned people." They may also have problems digesting milk and thus may avoid a major food source of vitamin D, he says.

Q: Are there problems with vitamin D toxicity?

A: High doses of vitamin D may cause too high levels of calcium in the blood. Symptoms include loss of appetite, nausea, vomiting, constipation and fatigue. High doses can also cause the buildup of calcium in soft tissue, such as muscles, which impairs their function. Most researchers agree that doses of less than 1,000 I.U. daily are unlikely to cause any adverse affects.

VITAMIN D
QUICK-REFERENCE GUIDE

RDA
For men and for women ages 11 to 24, 400 I.U.; for women age 25 and older, 200 I.U.

SOURCES
Fatty fish (such as mackerel, tuna and salmon), liver, egg yolks, fortified milk and cereals.

SIGNS OF DEFICIENCY
In children, bones so soft they develop curves when subjected to the body's weight. In adults, bone pain and tenderness, and muscle weakness.

POSSIBLE TOXICITY PROBLEMS
High doses of vitamin D may cause too high levels of calcium in the blood and calcium deposits in soft tissues. Symptoms include loss of appetite, nausea, vomiting, constipation and fatigue. Doses of less than 1,000 I.U. daily are unlikely to cause adverse affects.

VITAMIN E

Q: What is vitamin E?

A: Like vitamins A, D and K, vitamin E is a fat-soluble vitamin. It is a light yellow oil that comes in a variety of forms, both natural and synthetic. The most common naturally occurring forms are alpha-tocopherol and d-alpha-tocopherol. The most common synthetic forms are dl-alpha-tocopherol acetate and dl-alpha-tocopherol.

The natural forms are usually derived from soybean or wheat-germ oil, and the synthetic forms are manufactured from purified petroleum oil. Synthetic vitamin E forms have a bit less biological activity in the body than the natural forms, but researchers don't think that's a problem. It simply means you need a slightly larger amount of synthetic vitamin E than natural vitamin E to produce the same amount of biological activity.

Q: What is the RDA of vitamin E?

A: The RDA is 15 I.U. (10 mg.) of d-alpha-tocopherol or 10 tocopherol equivalents (TE) for men; for women, it's 12 I.U. (8 mg.) or 8 TE.

Q: What is a tocopherol equivalent?

A: It's an arbitrary unit of measurement that allows the different forms of vitamin E, all with varying levels of biological activity in the body, to be compared and measured. One tocopherol equivalent equals 1 milligram of d-alpha-tocopherol, which is also one I.U.

Q: What does vitamin E do?

A: Unlike other vitamins, which take part in metabolic reactions or function as hormones, vitamin E apparently has only one role—to act as an antioxidant.

That role, however, is an important one. The first vitamin discovered to act as an antioxidant, vitamin E is considered to be the strongest antioxidant. It works in concert with other antioxidants, especially with vitamin C and the trace mineral selenium, to provide antioxidant protection throughout the body.

Q: Didn't I read recently that vitamin E can protect against heart disease?

A: New research suggests that, yes, vitamin E has a significant impact on the development of heart disease.

Two large studies—one looking at women, the other at men—showed that vitamin E supplements substantially reduced the risk of heart disease. Conducted by researchers at Boston's Brigham and Women's Hospital and the Harvard School of Public Health, the studies found that people who took supplemental vitamin E every day had a 40 percent drop in heart-attack risk compared with those who did not take vitamin E supplements. The greatest protection was found at levels of about 100 I.U. of vitamin E a day for more than two years.

Q: How does vitamin E help prevent heart disease?

A: Its most important role may be helping to prevent the oxidation of artery-clogging LDL (low-density lipoprotein) cholesterol.

"It appears now that one of the earliest stages in the development of heart disease is the oxidation of LDL cholesterol," Dr. Blumberg says. LDL cholesterol is deposited on blood-vessel walls, where it is consumed by a certain type of immune cell, called a macrophage. Inside the cell, the LDL cholesterol becomes oxidized, and the macrophage turns into what's called a foam cell—a bloated, fat-laden cell. Heart disease begins as foam cells accumulate on blood-vessel walls, blocking the flow of blood through a vessel. By preventing the oxidation of LDL cholesterol, vitamin E prevents the formation of foam cells.

Q: So that's how it works?

A: Wait—there's more. Vitamin E also helps to prevent what's called **platelet aggregation**. Platelets are disk-shaped blood components that are involved in blood clotting. They can also clot up in blood vessels when they shouldn't. Getting adequate amounts of vitamin E prevents the platelets from clumping together and from sticking to blood-vessel walls.

Further, vitamin E can help prevent the tissue damage that can occur when blood is cut off then resupplied, as might happen in the case of a blood-vessel spasm or during surgery, when a blood vessel might be briefly clamped. Oxygen in the returning blood supply sets off a free-radical chain reaction that can damage tissue. Vitamin E helps keep free-radical damage to a minimum.

Q: What about cancer? Does vitamin E provide protection from cancer?

A: Although the correlation isn't as consistent as it is for vitamin C, numerous population studies show a link between vitamin E and cancer. People with the lowest blood levels of vitamin E tend to have the highest risks for certain cancers.

One study, by researchers at the National Cancer Institute Division of Cancer Etiology, recently found that people who took vitamin E as a separate supplement (100 I.U.) had half the risk of oral cancer of those who took no supplements or those who took multivitamins, which usually contain only 30 I.U. of vitamin E.

Q: How exactly is vitamin E supposed to help prevent cancer?

A: Experts think it works in at least three ways. First, by shielding a cell from free radicals, vitamin E prevents the kind of chromosome damage that can lead to cancer. "There is limited evidence that vitamin E can promote the repair of early chromosome damage," says Dr. Blumberg of the USDA Human Nutrition Research Center on Aging at Tufts University, in Boston. "And there is good evidence in animal studies that vitamin E slows the rate at which cells mutate and so may delay the onset of cancer for years."

Second, by combining with certain substances in the intestines, vitamin E can inhibit the formation of carcinogens— substances that can cause cell changes that lead to cancer. For instance, vitamin E helps stop the formation of cancer-promoting nitrosamines in the stomach. Nitrosamines are produced during the digestion of nitrates and nitrites, which are found in especially high concentration in preserved meats, such as hot dogs and bacon.

Third, by enhancing the body's immune response, vitamin E keeps the body's cancer "early surveillance system" in peak operating order. "Having adequate vitamin E in your blood means your immune cells are in a vigorous state, ready to attack the first cancer cells they see, which in fact is your primary defense against cancer," Dr. Blumberg explains.

Q: I've heard that vitamin E is supposed to do a lot of other things, too. Isn't it used to prevent breast tenderness, to reduce symptoms of premenstrual syndrome and to prevent scars from burns?

A: You're absolutely right. Vitamin E has been recommended and is used for all those things and more. But there aren't many studies substantiating its use for these health problems.

In a few studies, vitamin E seemed to provide some relief from fibrocystic breast changes, which can lead to multiple breast cysts. In one study, 22 of 26 women improved after taking 600 I.U. of vitamin E daily for eight weeks. But in another study, vitamin E provided no more relief than a placebo.

In two studies, 300 to 600 I.U. a day of vitamin E also seemed to help a number of premenstrual symptoms.

As for its ability to prevent scars, the medical world in general remains skeptical, although chances are you've heard a lot of people testify to the vitamin's benefits. "All that data is anecdotal," Dr. Blumberg says. "I know surgeons who swear by it, who tell their patients to apply it to their sutures. And hundreds of people have told me it just works miracles. But I know of no controlled clinical studies that demonstrate it makes wounds heal faster or prevents scarring."

Q: Is there anything else vitamin E is good for?

A: It is well established that vitamin E plays a crucial role in normal nerve function, and that a deficiency can contribute to nerve damage and some neurological disorders.

In a study done by Canadian researchers, vitamin E helped reduce the number of epileptic seizures in children. And vitamin E has proved useful in a neurological disorder called tardive dyskinesia, which is a side effect of long-term use of tranquilizers prescribed to curb psychotic behavior.

Supplemental doses of vitamin E appear to boost immune-system function in older people, to help people with noninsulin-dependent diabetes maintain metabolic control, to ease mouth sores in people receiving cancer chemotherapy and, in older people, to minimize free-radical-induced muscle damage associated with hard use.

Q: You didn't mention sex. Isn't vitamin E supposed to increase sexual prowess?

A: Claims that vitamin E increases sex drive in both men and women abound, but there is no evidence to support these claims.

Q: Do people ever take much larger doses than the RDA of vitamin E?

A: Yes, doses of 100, 400, even 800 I.U. have been suggested, and in studies where benefits have been noted, the amount of vitamin E used has exceeded the RDA.

Q: Any proof that these larger doses could be harmful?

A: For the most part, vitamin E is considered to be quite safe, even in large amounts. Researchers for the Brigham and Harvard study noted, though, that amounts higher than 100 to 400 I.U. did not further reduce the risk of heart disease, because intakes higher than 400 I.U. do not further increase blood levels of the vitamin.

Q: What are the best sources of vitamin E?

A: Hazelnut oil, wheat-germ oil, sunflower oil, almond oil, wheat germ, mayonnaise, whole-grain cereals and eggs are all good sources.

However, a recent study by researchers at the University of California, in Berkeley, found that people are most likely to get their vitamin E from mayonnaise and salad dressing; margarine; doughnuts, cookies and cake; french fries and fried potatoes; salad and cooking oils; pies and eggs.

That study also found that one of the biggest contributors of vitamin E is superfortified cereals, such as Total and Product 19, that contain the RDA of vitamin E. Only a small percentage of people eat such cereals, according to this study.

Q: Do people get enough vitamin E?

A: This study found that most people did not reach the RDA. Men were consuming 7.3 mg. TE and women 5.4 mg. TE of vitamin E a day. That's less than the RDA. Elderly and poor people were likely to get even less.

What's more, there is "absolutely no way" you can get the large doses of vitamin E used in clinical trials through your diet, says Dr. Blumberg. "You may be able to get 15 to 30 I.U. a day through diet, and people who try really hard and eat lots of nuts and margarine might get up to 40 to 50 I.U. But that's about as high as anyone can go by diet alone," he stresses. So supplements are necessary to reach high levels.

Q: Are people likely to develop a vitamin E deficiency?

A: No. Even though they may be lower in vitamin E than might be wise in terms of chronic-disease prevention, most people do not develop vitamin E-deficiency symptoms. It's hard to induce such symptoms in animals; indeed, symptoms are uncommon even in Third World countries.

Q: Who is likely to develop a vitamin E deficiency?

A: As we said, vitamin E deficiency is not commonly found. Those who are at higher risk of developing it, however, include people who, for a variety of reasons, do not absorb fat normally; premature, very low birthweight infants; older people; people on very-low-fat diets; and people with chronic liver disease or cystic fibrosis.

Q: What are the signs of deficiency?

A: In infants, irritability, fluid retention and anemia. In adults, lethargy, apathy, inability to concentrate, ataxia (staggering gait, loss of balance) and anemia.

Q: What do I need to know about taking vitamin E supplements?

A: Most vitamin E supplements are available as 200 or 400 I.U. oil-filled capsules. Don't take vitamin E supplements without your doctor's okay if you're taking anticoagulant drugs.

It's also well known that the more vegetable oils you consume, the higher your need for vitamin E. That's because polyunsaturated fats—contained in many vegetable oils— are easily oxidized in the body. As people switch from animal products to vegetable oils, their vitamin E requirement may double.

Further, even though vegetable oils are generally considered a good source of vitamin E, a University of California at Berkeley study found that even people consuming large amounts of vegetable oils did not have what is considered an adequate ratio of polyunsaturated fats to vitamin E. And refined vegetable oils, such as corn oil or olive oil, are not good sources of vitamin E, Dr. Blumberg says. "In fact, natural-source vitamin supplements are made from the stuff that's *removed* during processing from commercial vegetable oils such as soybean oil."

VITAMIN E
QUICK-REFERENCE GUIDE

RDA
For men, 15 I.U. or 10 mg. TE; for women, 12 I.U. or 8 mg. TE.

SOURCES
Hazelnut oil, wheat-germ oil, sunflower oil, almond oil, wheat germ, mayonnaise, whole-grain cereals, eggs and fortified cereals.

SIGNS OF DEFICIENCY
In infants, irritability, fluid retention and anemia. In adults, lethargy, apathy, inability to concentrate, loss of balance, staggering gait, and anemia.

POSSIBLE TOXICITY PROBLEMS
Toxicity is considered low. The Food and Nutrition Board concedes that there is little evidence of harm at doses of less than 1,000 I.U. per day.

VITAMIN K

Q: I know you mentioned it before, but does vitamin K actually exist?

A: It's true that the letter labeling for vitamins does skip a few characters right after E. But don't let that fool you. Vitamin K is for real, although it's probably one of the least known fat-soluble vitamins. It was assigned an RDA as recently as 1989. A yellow oil or crystal in its pure form, only its natural form is used for humans. Like vitamins A, D and E, vitamin K is fat-soluble.

Q: What is the RDA for vitamin K?

A: It is very low—for men, 80 mcg. per day, the amount found in about one-half cup cooked cabbage or less than one-half cup broccoli. For women, the RDA is 65 mcg.

Q: What does vitamin K do in the body?

A: The researchers who discovered this nutrient labeled it K for koagulation—in Danish, anyway. Vitamin K is used in the liver to manufacture at least four different proteins important in blood clotting. Without this nutrient, a simple cut or scrape could leave you spilling blood all over the floor.

Q: Does this mean that if I am deficient in this vitamin, I'll bleed easily or for a long time?

A: Yes, that is a sign of deficiency. In fact, doctors check for vitamin K deficiency with a test that measures how long it takes a person's blood to clot—called prothrombin time. But keep in mind that there are other things besides a vitamin K deficiency that can interfere with blood clotting.

Q: Does vitamin K do anything besides clot blood?

A: This vitamin is also involved in the production of two other proteins, one related to bone metabolism, the other to kidney function, says James Sadowski, Ph.D., chief of the vitamin K laboratory at the Human Nutrition Research Center on Aging at Tufts University, in Boston. "We're not yet sure just how a vitamin K deficiency may affect these organs, though," he says.

In a study by Dutch researchers, large supplemental doses of 1 mg. a day of vitamin K seemed to improve the calcium status of postmenopausal women. It boosted blood levels of a calcium-carrying protein, osteocalcin, thought to be involved in bone building. It also decreased calcium excretion through the urine.

Q: Who is likely to be at risk for deficiency?

A: Vitamin K deficiency is not common. It seems to occur most frequently in people with impaired fat absorption, people who have prolonged diarrhea, or seriously ill persons. It can also occur in newborn and premature babies.

Q: What happens with people who are seriously ill?

A: The typical—and occasionally fatal—scenario includes a person in the hospital who is being given antibiotics to prevent or overcome infections and who is being fed a formula diet that does not include vitamin K. The antibiotics have killed his intestinal bacteria, which normally can synthesize some vitamin K. Thus, his vitamin K stores are depleted. He may develop stomach or intestinal bleeding, or, if he undergoes surgery, he may bleed to death. That's why clotting time should always be checked before surgery.

Q: How are these people treated?

A: These people often require injections or dietary supplements of this nutrient until clotting time returns to normal, according to Dr. Sadowski.

Q: If clotting time is affected by a deficiency in vitamin K, what about people taking blood thinners?

A: Vitamin K supplements aren't usually given to people taking blood-thinning (anticoagulant) drugs, since they counteract the effect of these drugs, Dr. Sadowksi says. In fact, getting too much vitamin K in your diet may be one reason these drugs are sometimes hard to regulate. People taking blood-thinning drugs may do well to keep their intake of vitamin K-rich foods constant so that their dosage of blood thinner remains effective, experts say.

Q: You mentioned newborn and premature babies. Why are they deficient in vitamin K? Do they have bleeding problems because of this? What's done about it?

A: "Babies apparently are low in vitamin K because this vitamin is not easily transferred from mother to baby," explains Walter J. Morales, M.D., Ph.D., director of maternal/fetal medicine at Arnold Palmer Hospital for Women and Children, in Orlando, Florida. Only if a mother gets a large amount of vitamin K (from injections) does it cross the placental barrier to provide protection to the baby. Newborn babies are given a vitamin K shot soon after they reach the nursery, a practice that has dramatically reduced deaths from brain hemorrhage after birth, according to Dr. Morales.

Q: But what about premature babies?

A: Premature babies run a high risk of brain hemorrhage during delivery, because their blood vessels are too fragile to withstand the surges in blood pressure that occur during delivery. That's why some doctors now give vitamin K shots to women at high risk of delivering premature babies.

In a study conducted by Dr. Morales, brain hemorrhaging occurred in only 11 percent of the babies of mothers who got such injections, compared with 36 percent of babies of mothers who did not receive injections. And none of the babies who received vitamin K via their mothers had severe brain hemorrhaging.

"Since there are no side effects to this treatment, we err on the side of safety," Dr. Morales says. He uses vitamin K in any pregnancy expected to result in delivery at 30 weeks or less. He administers vitamin K at least five hours prior to estimated delivery to make sure it has time to cross the placenta into the baby's blood.

Q: What foods are good sources of vitamin K?

A: Dark, leafy greens offer the most vitamin K. Kale has about 1,000 mcg. per cup, spinach, about 630 mcg., and turnip greens, 440 mcg. Two tablespoons of fresh chopped parsley has about 7 mcg.

Broccoli, brussels sprouts, Chinese cabbage, lettuce and watercress are also good sources. Cabbage, carrots, avocados, cucumbers, leeks, tomatoes and dairy products are fair sources.

Oils made from green plants are also a good source: Olive, canola and soybean oils fit that bill. Meats and cereals also contain some vitamin K.

A variety of foods, such as dairy products, vegetable oils,

meats and cereals, offer a bit of vitamin K. Consequently, experts agree that, even if people don't eat the foods that are excellent sources of this nutrient, they still get enough of it.

Q: Is vitamin K available as a supplement?

A: You may find it in some of the higher-priced multivitamins. It's usually listed on the label as **phylloquinone**, its natural form.

But single-nutrient supplements are available only by prescription. For those at risk for deficiency, supplementation with 50 to 100 mcg. daily is considered safe and desirable, experts say. They add that even though the risk for toxicity from vitamin K is low, people with a vitamin K deficiency should be treated by a doctor.

VITAMIN K
QUICK-REFERENCE GUIDE

RDA
For men, 80 mcg.; for women, 65 mcg.

SOURCES
Dark, leafy greens, such as kale, spinach, and parsley; broccoli, brussels sprouts, Chinese cabbage, lettuce, watercress, carrots, avocados, cucumbers and leeks; olive, canola and soybean oils. Meats and cereals also contain some vitamin K.

SIGNS OF DEFICIENCY
Prolonged clotting time, easy bleeding and bruising, frequent nosebleeds.

POSSIBLE TOXICITY PROBLEMS
Large amounts from foods or supplements can interfere with the action of blood-thinning drugs.

---

9 MINERALS

CALCIUM

Q: What is calcium?

A: Calcium is a silvery-white metallic element found in such common substances as chalk, granite, eggshell, seashells, hard water, bone and limestone. The body of a 150-pound adult contains about three pounds of calcium, making it the most abundant mineral in the body.

Q: In what foods is calcium found?

A: Milk and dairy products, such as cheese and ice cream, are the richest sources. Kale, turnip greens, kelp, tofu, canned salmon and sardines (with bones), and soybeans are good sources, but most people in the United States do not eat these foods in large enough quantities to meet calcium's 800 mg. RDA.

Q: What role does calcium play in the body?

A: Building of bones and teeth is calcium's most familiar role. Some 99 percent of the body's calcium is found in bones or teeth. However, calcium is also essential for nerve conduction, muscle contraction, heartbeat, blood clotting, the production of energy and the maintenance of immune function, among other things.

Q: Does calcium keep bones and teeth hard?

A: Yes. It's not the only mineral involved in this process, but it is an important one. Bone consists of cells and fiber embedded in a mineral matrix, mostly crystals of calcium phosphate, along with magnesium, sodium and trace minerals. And bone undergoes changes throughout life. It's possible for your body to draw calcium from your bones to maintain adequate levels in your bloodstream. And calcium can be delivered to bones throughout your lifetime, too, although the body is most efficient at making bone up to age 30. After that, bone density tends to slack off.

Q: Yes, I've heard that people's bones get weaker as they age. Can getting enough calcium throughout my lifetime prevent that from happening?

A: The condition you're referring to is osteoporosis—literally, porous bones. Some people, especially postmenopausal women, develop such severe osteoporosis that their bones break under their bodies' own weight.

Research shows that getting enough calcium early in life, up to age 30, can help prevent osteoporosis by allowing bones to reach their maximum density. Then, when bones lose density later in life, they are less likely to become so weak that they fracture.

Q: What about calcium supplementation later in life?

A: Some research also shows that getting large amounts of calcium later in life helps to slow the bone loss associated with osteoporosis. In one study of postmenopausal women, a calcium supplement of 1,000 mg. a day reduced the loss of bone mineral density by 43 percent when compared with a group receiving a placebo. The rate of bone loss in the legs was reduced by 35 percent, and, in the spine, bone loss was stopped. That's an important finding, because many of the fractures associated with osteoporosis are tiny breaks in the spinal vertebrae.

In another study, women taking a combination of 1,200 mg. of calcium and 20 mcg. of vitamin D had a 70 percent reduction in the risk of hip fractures after 18 months of supplementation.

Q: I've heard that getting extra calcium in your diet can help prevent muscle cramps, including menstrual cramps. Is that true?

A: Calcium is involved in the process of muscle contraction and relaxation, and a calcium deficiency can lead to severe muscle spasms. Obstetricians occasionally prescribe extra calcium to pregnant women who complain of leg cramps, and one study showed that calcium supplementation helped reduce the incidence of leg cramps in pregnant women.

Calcium, along with magnesium, is sometimes recommended to relieve both menstrual cramps and symptoms associated with premenstrual syndrome. One recent study by USDA researchers suggests that calcium actually can relieve some of these symptoms. In that study, women getting 1,300 mg. of calcium a day reported fewer problems with mood swings or ability to concentrate than women getting only 600 mg. of calcium. The women getting extra calcium also reported fewer aches and pains during menstruation.

Q: Isn't there some research showing that calcium helps to prevent colon cancer?

A: Several studies indicate that people getting lots of calcium in their diets are less likely to develop colon cancer than those getting only small amounts. From these studies, it appears that men getting the calcium equivalent of about 1½ cups of milk a day have three times the risk of developing colon or rectal cancer than men getting calcium equal to 4½ cups of milk a day.

Q: How does calcium prevent colon cancer?

A: Calcium can bind with cancer-promoting bile acids produced in the colon, which reduces intestinal irritation. And in test tubes, calcium is able to normalize the growth of cells lining the intestinal wall, so it is able to inhibit the kind of cell growth that could lead to cancer. Several studies are in progress to see if large amounts of calcium—up to three grams a day—can reduce the development of potentially cancerous intestinal polyps in people at high risk for colon cancer.

Q: Is calcium helpful for anything else?

A: In several studies, calcium supplementation has provided a modest reduction in blood pressure— about five points—in people with established hypertension, or high blood pressure. And in one study, people who consumed at least 1,000 mg. of calcium a day—the equivalent of three servings of dairy products—reduced their risk of high blood pressure by about 12 percent. In that study, people who got the most benefit from a high-calcium diet were those age 40 or younger, thin people and those having no more than one alcoholic drink a day. (Alcohol depletes the body of calcium.)

If it's given both before and during pregnancy, calcium can also prevent pregnancy-induced hypertension, a condition dangerous to both mother and fetus. A daily two-gram dose of calcium lowered the risk of pregnancy-induced hypertension to 10 percent, compared with 15 percent in a group of women receiving a placebo.

Adequate calcium intake can also protect people exposed to lead, experts say. Lead absorption is blocked by calcium in the intestines.

Q: How much calcium do most people get each day?

A: Men do better than women, since their higher-calorie diets provide more of most minerals. Studies indicate that about 10 percent of people get less than 50 percent of the RDA of calcium. Some 60 percent of women ages 35 to 74 get less than two-thirds of the RDA.

Q: Is more than the RDA of calcium ever recommended?

A: Yes. In 1984, a special panel of the National Institutes of Health made these recommendations: premenopausal women: 1,000 mg. calcium daily; postmenopausal women not taking estrogen replacement: 1,500 mg. calcium daily; postmenopausal women taking estrogen: 1,000 mg. calcium daily.

Q: What are signs of calcium deficiency?

A: Signs of calcium deficiency include abnormal heartbeat; muscle pains and cramps; numbness; stiffness and tingling of the hands and feet; and dementia.

Q: Who's likely to be calcium-deficient?

A: People who avoid dairy products, along with those consuming low-calorie, high-protein or high-fiber diets; people who drink a lot of alcohol; and users of aluminum-containing antacids, which inhibit calcium absorption.

Q: I've heard that drinking lots of milk can make a person develop kidney stones. Is that true?

A: No. Kidney stones used to be considered a possible side effect of a high-calcium diet, because most kidney stones do contain calcium. But a recent study showed that men getting the most calcium in their diets had only one-third the risk of developing kidney stones compared with men eating low-calcium diets. A high-calcium diet makes you excrete oxalate, a component of kidney stones that may prove to be more important than calcium, researchers say.

CALCIUM
QUICK-REFERENCE GUIDE

RDA
800 mg. for men and women. The National Institutes of Health has made these special recommendations: premenopausal women: 1,000 mg. calcium daily; postmenopausal women not taking estrogen replacement: 1,500 mg. calcium daily; post-menopausal women taking estrogen: 1,000 mg. calcium daily.

SOURCES
Milk and dairy products (such as cheese and ice cream), kale, turnip greens, kelp, tofu, canned salmon and sardines (with bones) and soybeans.

SIGNS OF DEFICIENCY
Abnormal heartbeat, muscle pains and cramps, numbness, stiffness and tingling of the hands and feet, dementia.

POSSIBLE TOXICITY PROBLEMS
Doses up to 2,500 mg. a day are considered safe. Gastrointestinal complaints such as nausea, gas and constipation can be avoided by taking divided doses with meals, or sticking with calcium gluconate or calcium lactate, the two most soluble forms. Early signs of high blood calcium—vomiting, nausea, loss of appetite—occur only in people who have taken enormous doses of 25,000 mg. or more. High blood levels of calcium rarely happens as a result of calcium intake alone.

CHROMIUM

Q: What is chromium?

A: Chromium is an essential trace mineral, and the same metal that's used to make the shiny chrome-plated bumpers on cars.

Q: In what foods is chromium found?

A: The richest known sources are liver, brewer's yeast and certain spices, such as black pepper and thyme. Beef, poultry, broccoli, whole-grain cereals, bran, wheat germ and oysters are also good sources.

Q: What role does chromium play in the body?

A: The body needs chromium to be able to burn sugar for energy, a process called glucose metabolism. People with hypoglycemia, or low blood sugar, or with a condition called insulin resistance show improved glucose metabolism when given 250 mcg. of chromium. This helps to keep blood-sugar levels stable, and so, helps prevent damage to blood vessels and organs, such as the heart and kidney, caused by high levels of blood sugar.

In the body, chromium becomes part of an enzyme called glucose tolerance factor. This compound enhances the body's response to insulin, helping move glucose into cells where it can be burned for energy. Glucose tolerance factor is also found in brewer's yeast and is considered the most biologically active and absorbable form of chromium.

Q: Does that mean that getting adequate chromium in my diet can prevent diabetes?

A: So far, there is no direct evidence that chromium helps prevent diabetes, or that it helps lessen established diabetes. Nevertheless, insulin resistance and hypoglycemia are often early signs of diabetes, and chromium has been proven to help both of these conditions.

Q: Anything else chromium is good for?

A: In one study, supplementation with 250 mcg. a day of chromium-improved blood-cholesterol levels, raising heart-healthy HDL cholesterol and lowering triglycerides.

And in a study that has yet to be duplicated, a laboratory-concocted form of chromium, called chromium picolinate, extended the lifespan of rats by one year. That may not seem like much, but it is a gain of 36 percent in the normal lifespan of a rat—the equivalent of a man or woman living to be 110. In these rats, blood sugar and hemoglobin remained lower in the chromium-supplemented rats when compared with a control group. The researchers speculate that chromium supplementation provides some of the same glucose-lowering benefits as calorie restriction by eliminating degenerative diseases such as kidney and heart disease. Calorie restriction is the only method so far that in laboratory experiments has been proven to consistently extend lifespan in animals.

Chromium picolinate is available as a supplement.

Q: Do people get enough chromium in their diets?

A: Chromium intake from the typical American diet is estimated at less than 50 micrograms a day, an amount far below that found beneficial in studies, and at the lower edge of the adequate range. Refined grains and oils require chromium to be metabolized but contain no chromium. So they deplete the body of this nutrient.

CHROMIUM
QUICK-REFERENCE GUIDE

RDA
No RDA, but an Estimated Safe and Adequate Daily Intake is 50 to 200 mcg. a day for both men and women.

SOURCES
Liver, brewer's yeast, black pepper, thyme, beef, poultry, broccoli, whole-grain cereals, bran, wheat germ and oysters.

SIGNS OF DEFICIENCY
Glucose intolerance, weight loss, diabetes-like symptoms, nerve degeneration.

POSSIBLE TOXICITY PROBLEMS
Little is known about the possible toxic effects of chromium, including how much is too much. Biologically active forms of chromium, such as glucose tolerance factor, found in brewer's yeast, and chromium picolinate, are much better absorbed than chromium chloride, the kind most often found in supplements.

While people with diabetes may benefit from chromium supplementation, their insulin requirements may change as a result. So their use of supplements should be monitored by a doctor.

COPPER

Q: What is copper?

A: Copper is an essential trace mineral. It's the brownish metal that once was used to make pennies. (Now they're mostly zinc.) In the body, copper combines with proteins or with other metals, such as iron or zinc, to make chemical compounds that have biological activity.

Q: In what foods is copper found?

A: The best sources are beef or chicken livers, crabs, nuts, seeds, peanut butter, fruit, oysters, kidneys and beans.

Q: What role does copper play in the body?

A: Like iron, copper is necessary for the formation of red blood cells, and also helps to carry and store iron. It's necessary for the formation of collagen, the connective tissue used to form bone, cartilage, skin and tendons. It helps produce melanin, a pigment that gives color to skin and hair. (In animals, loss of fur pigmentation is a sign of copper deficiency.)

Copper also acts as an antioxidant and anti-inflammatory in the body, and there is some evidence that it helps to prevent heart disease and cancer.

Q: Wow. That's a lot. Let's start with blood formation. Does copper deficiency cause anemia the way iron deficiency does?

A: Yes, because iron needs copper to form hemoglobin, the oxygen-carrying protein in the blood, copper deficiency can lead to a type of anemia that is very similar to iron-deficiency anemia, explains Leslie Klevay, M.D., a researcher at the USDA Human Nutrition Research Center, in Grand Forks, North Dakota. Copper-deficiency anemia isn't often diagnosed, however, perhaps because it is mistaken for iron-deficiency anemia, or perhaps because the two may occur concurrently. It has been noted since the 1920s that iron-deficiency anemia resolves more quickly if both iron and copper are given.

Q: If copper is necessary for the formation of connective tissue, what happens to bones and skin and other tissues if there is not enough copper?

A: In animals, copper deficiency leads to all sorts of blood-vessel and bone defects, including aneurysms (weakening of the blood-vessel walls that can lead to blow-outs), rupture of the heart, hemorrhaging of the surface of bones, and bone fractures. It can also cause lung disorders, faulty wool or hair structure, degeneration of the nervous system, heart disease and internal hemorrhaging. In humans, copper deficiency has been linked with bone fractures and hemorrhage, and weakness of the blood-vessel walls, including some types of aneurysms.

Q: What about cancer? You said copper may help prevent cancer.

A: There is no direct evidence that supplemental copper can protect humans from cancer. Several animal studies, however, suggest that copper may help protect against cancer. In one study, supplementary copper in the diets of rats protected them from chemical-caused cancer. In another, copper protected chicks against a type of virus-induced cancer. The speculation is that copper, like vitamins C and E, works as an antioxidant to neutralize free radicals involved in cancer-promoting processes. Copper is part of an important antioxidant enzyme, copper-zinc superoxide dismutase, as well as the antioxidant called ceruloplasmin, which has both antioxidant and anti-inflammatory properties and may play a role in the body's reaction to such inflammatory conditions as rheumatoid arthritis.

Q: And heart disease? How is copper involved in that?

A: Copper deficiencies have been associated with unfavorable changes in blood fats, a significant drop in heart-healthy HDL cholesterol and, in some studies, an increase in artery-clogging LDL cholesterol, according to research done by Dr. Klevay. In animals, low copper intake has also been associated with weakening and rupture of the heart muscle.

Q: Hasn't copper somehow been associated with rheumatoid arthritis?

A: People with rheumatoid arthritis sometimes resort to wearing copper bracelets in an attempt to relieve their symptoms, but the connection between copper status and this type of inflammatory arthritis remains unclear, says Mark Failla, Ph.D., a professor of human nutrition at the University of North Carolina at Greensboro.

What is known is that during inflammation or infection, two copper-containing enzymes, superoxide dismutase and ceruloplasmin, are mobilized in the body. In people with rheumatoid arthritis, for instance, ceruloplasmin levels are elevated two to three times. Levels also go up in the fluid within inflamed joints.

This has led researchers to speculate that ceruloplasm has an important function in helping minimize damage associated with chronic inflammatory conditions, such as rheumatoid arthritis, Dr. Failla says.

However, the precise connection remains unclear, since people with rheumatoid arthritis do not appear to be deficient in copper. "It's possible some people with rheumatoid arthritis do have a higher copper requirement than normal," according to Dr. Failla. He and other copper researchers suggest you eat plenty of copper-containing foods, or that you take multivitamin and mineral tablets containing two mg. of copper.

Q: Do people get enough copper in their diets?

A: Dietary surveys show that about one-third of people get less than 1 mg. a day of copper, and that about two-thirds of people get less than 1.5 mg., which is the lower limit of the suggested amount for adults.

Q: What are signs of deficiency?

A: Symptoms include anemia, paleness, bone and connective-tissue problems, disorders of blood-fat metabolism, "steel wool" hair, internal hemorrhaging, problems with temperature regulation, convulsions, impaired glucose tolerance, increased blood pressure and heartbeat problems.

COPPER
QUICK-REFERENCE GUIDE

RDA
No RDA, but an Estimated Safe and Adequate Daily Intake of copper for adults is 1.5 to 3 mg.

SOURCES
Beef or chicken liver; crab; chocolate; sunflower, sesame and poppy seeds; nuts; peanut butter; fruit; oysters; kidneys and beans.

SIGNS OF DEFICIENCY
Anemia, paleness, bone and connective-tissue disorders, disorders of blood-fat metabolism, "steel wool" hair, internal hemorrhaging, problems with temperature regulation, convulsions, impaired glucose tolerance, increased blood pressure, heartbeat problems.

POSSIBLE TOXICITY PROBLEMS
Experts say that occasional intake of up to 10 mg. a day is safe, but that copper intake over extended periods of time should be in the range of 2 to 3 mg. a day. People with Wilson's disease, a genetic condition marked by overaccumulation of copper, should not take copper supplements.

IODINE

Q: What is iodine?

A: Iodine is a nonmetallic, blackish-gray element that is essential for good health. When it is isolated under laboratory conditions, iodine is a gas. However, in nature, it is found only as a compound and as a liquid or solid.

Q: In what foods is iodine found?

A: Rich sources include seaweeds (such as kelp), fish, shrimp, lobster, clams, oysters, the thyroid glands of animals (sweet breads) and iodized salt.

Q: What role does iodine play in the body?

A: Iodine is necessary for the formation of two hormones produced by the thyroid gland, the largest of the endocrine glands in the body, located in the front and sides of the neck around the windpipe. The thyroid gland produces hormones that are vital for growth, reproduction, nerve formation and mental health, bone formation, the manufacture of proteins, and a cell's oxidative processes. These hormones serve as the major regulators of energy metabolism in the body.

Q: What are signs of iodine deficiency?

A: Symptoms include chronic fatigue, apathy, dry skin, intolerance to cold, weight gain and enlargement of the thyroid, a condition known as goiter that used to be fairly common in the United States before fortification of salt with iodine was instituted in the 1920s.

Q: **Is iodine used to treat any diseases?**

A: Of course, iodine is used to treat goiter. Iodine can also be used to prevent radiation damage to the thyroid gland.

Q: **Radiation damage? From x-rays?**

A: No, from a nuclear accident or in the event of nuclear war. Radioactive compounds—iodides—are released into the environment following such events. They can enter the body and accumulate in the thyroid gland, where they remain for varying periods of time. Radioactive iodine can cause thyroid cancer. However, loading up the thyroid gland with nonradioactive iodine prior to or as soon as possible after a nuclear accident can reduce radioiodine uptake by the thyroid to practically zero.

Q: **Is iodine used for any other health problems?**

A: Some researchers believe that fibrocystic problems of the breast—painful swelling and lumpiness prior to menstruation—are the result of iodine deficiency. And one Canadian study found that the majority of women with painful, lumpy breasts experienced complete relief from their symptoms after being treated with iodine for four months. Most doctors, however, believe more research needs to be done in this area before iodine can be recommended for this problem.

Some iodine-containing compounds, such as supersaturated potassium iodide, are helpful in breaking up clogged mucus in breathing tubes. These are drugs that require a doctor's prescription.

Iodine is also an antiseptic. Iodine-containing tablets are frequently used by hikers to disinfect water.

Q: Any problems with toxicity?

A: Different forms of iodine have different levels of toxicity. Elemental iodine—the kind that's sold as an antiseptic—is quite toxic. People have died from ingesting less than two grams of elemental iodine. Supplements contain a less toxic form, usually potassium iodide, either by itself or in combination with other vitamins and minerals. Taking several milligrams of any kind of iodine can cause thyroid problems or inflammation of the salivary glands.

Q: Who is likely to be deficient in iodine?

A: In the United States, iodine deficiency is rare. That's because people eat so much salt, and most salt is fortified with iodine. However, people who restrict their salt intake and who do not eat seafood may benefit from iodine supplementation.

IODINE
QUICK-REFERENCE GUIDE

RDA
For men and women, 150 mcg.

SOURCES
Kelp, fish, shrimp, lobster, clams, oysters, the thyroid glands of animals (sweet breads), and iodized salt.

SIGNS OF DEFICIENCY
Chronic fatigue, apathy, dry skin, intolerance to cold, weight gain and enlargement of the thyroid.

POSSIBLE TOXICITY PROBLEMS
Elemental iodine—the kind that's used as an antiseptic—can be deadly even in amounts as small as 2 grams. Several milligrams daily of iodine compounds have been linked with thyroid problems or inflammation of the salivary glands.

IRON

Q: What is iron?

A: Iron is the major element on earth, making up 35 percent of the earth's interior. Iron and its alloys, such as steel, are familiar substances to everyone. In the body, iron is involved in energy production and other important functions.

Q: In what foods is iron found?

A: Good sources of iron are liver, meats, beans, nuts, dried fruits, poultry, fish, whole grains or enriched cereals, and most dark green leafy vegetables. About 25 percent of the iron people get each day is from enriched foods.

Q: What role does iron play in the body?

A: Iron carries oxygen throughout the body. Since oxygen is required in every cell to produce energy, iron is the backbone of energy production. Iron is a part of hemoglobin, a protein that carries oxygen in red blood cells. It is also part of oxygen-carrying proteins in the muscles. Iron is involved in the production of thyroid hormones (which regulate many metabolic processes), in the production of connective tissues, in the maintenance of the immune system and in the production and regulation of several brain neurotransmitters. Low levels of iron have been linked with anemia, fatigue, rapid heartbeat, breathlessness, inability to concentrate, disturbed sleep, severe menstrual pain and bleeding, and hair loss.

Q: I thought you said earlier that oxygen was harmful to the body, but now you're telling me that it is an important part of energy production. What's the deal?

A: Oxidative reactions are vital for life, but can be harmful if they go beyond what is necessary for energy production. So iron does have its dark side. Oxygen can generate harmful free radicals, which, you'll recall, can damage cells by stealing electrons. Too much iron in the body means too much oxygen available to generate free radical damage.

Q: How do you end up with too much iron in your blood?

A: Several conditions are characterized by an excess of iron in the body. One condition, called **hemochromatosis**, is a genetic disorder, diagnosed in about 1 percent of people, in which there are excessive deposits of iron in the liver, heart, pancreas, skin and other organs, all of which are subject to serious damage from free radicals generated by the iron. Hemochromatosis is considered to be fairly rare, but some researchers think it is simply underdiagnosed. A simple blood test to check for this condition measures serum ferritin, the stored form of iron.

Q: Can you get too much iron from supplements or from eating iron-rich foods?

A: If you have hemochromatosis, getting too much iron from supplements, iron-enriched foods or even iron-rich foods can become a problem. However, normal people don't usually develop high levels of iron, because their intestines absorb less and less of it as iron levels reach optimum amounts in the blood.

Q: Has too much iron been associated with any health problems?

A: One study from Finland suggests that even as small as a 1 percent increase in iron levels can cause a 4 percent increase in risk for a heart attack. Most scientists, however, believe it is too soon to draw any definitive conclusions about iron's effects on the risk of heart disease.

Q: How would high iron levels contribute to heart disease?

A: Researchers think high levels of iron cause increased oxidative damage to the heart and blood vessels and, perhaps, increased oxidation of LDL cholesterol, which then begins to clog arteries.

Q: What about cancer? Are high iron levels associated with an increase in cancer?

A: Animal studies suggest that, depending on the conditions, iron can either enhance or inhibit tumor development. Iron is necessary for the division of cells, and, in some animals, iron deficiency has been shown to slow tumor growth. On the other hand, in population studies, iron deficiency has been associated with an increased risk for cancers of the throat and stomach. Research is going on right now to see if higher-than-normal body stores of iron increase a woman's risk of developing breast cancer.

Q: Have low iron levels been associated with any diseases?

A: Low levels of iron result in iron-deficiency anemia, a condition characterized by small, pale red blood cells and extreme fatigue, trouble concentrating, breathlessness and other problems. Simply increasing iron intake eventually corrects this problem, although some people initially need to take large amounts of iron to get back to normal.

Iron deficiency has also been associated with Plummer-Vinson syndrome. In this condition, a thin weblike membrane grows across the top of the esophagus, making it difficult to swallow. This syndrome used to be fairly common in Sweden but has been practically eliminated with the use of iron supplements.

Q: **I've heard that low iron intake can affect your mood and ability to concentrate and learn. Is that true?**

A: Yes. Iron-deficiency anemia has been implicated in emotional, social and learning difficulties in children and adults. Iron-deficient babies are often irritable and lack interest in their surroundings, and adults lacking iron are often sluggish and fuzzy-headed.

A recent study showed that both iron and copper deficiencies may interfere with a good night's sleep. People eating too little iron slept longer but woke more often during the night than those getting adequate amounts.

Another study showed that 105 mg. a day of supplemental iron helped stabilize mood swings, ability to concentrate in school and fatigue in teenage girls who'd complained about such symptoms.

Low iron levels may also increase the risk of several menstrual symptoms, including behavioral changes and autonomic sensations (such as sweating and dizziness), decreased efficiency, poor performance at work or school and increased daytime napping.

Q: **Is iron deficiency associated with any other problems?**

A: Immune response—the body's ability to fight off infection—drops off in people who are iron deficient. Both chronic yeast infections and herpes simplex infections are more common in people who are low on iron. Certain types of immune cells rely on iron to generate the oxidative reactions that allow these cells to kill off bacteria and other harmful invaders. When iron levels are low, these cells can't do their job properly.

Q: Don't some athletes take extra iron to boost their performance?

A: Unless you are running low on iron, extra amounts of this mineral do nothing to improve athletic performance. Iron deficiency is associated with muscle weakness and reduced stamina, however, and this weakness and loss of stamina apparently can occur even though iron levels have not dropped low enough to cause anemia. Studies in women suggest that moderate exercise does not deplete iron stores.

Q: Do most people get enough iron?

A: No. Dietary surveys show that many people don't get enough iron to meet their needs, with 32 percent of people getting less than 70 percent of the RDA of 10 mg. for men and postmenopausal women, and 15 mg. for premenopausal women. Iron deficiency is the most common nutritional deficiency in the United States.

Q: Who is most likely to be deficient in iron?

A: Infants, children and teenagers, especially girls, are often deficient, since rapid growth imposes a great need for iron. Deficiencies are also common in women during the childbearing years, since menstruation, pregnancy and lactation all draw on the body's iron stores.

IRON
QUICK-REFERENCE GUIDE

RDA
For men and for women age 50 or older, 10 mg.; for women
ages 11 to 50, 15 mg.

SOURCES
Liver, meats, beans, nuts, dried fruits, poultry, fish, whole grains
or enriched cereals, and most dark green leafy vegetables.

SIGNS OF DEFICIENCY
Anemia, fatigue, rapid heartbeat, breathlessness, inability to
concentrate, disturbed sleep, severe menstrual pain and
bleeding, and hair loss.

POSSIBLE TOXICITY PROBLEMS
Constipation is the most common side effect associated with
iron supplements. Children who take many tablets of iron-
containing supplements may end up in a hospital emergency
room, as large doses are poisonous to them. However, advances
in treatment have virtually eliminated childhood deaths from
iron poisoning. High body levels of iron may be associated
with an increased risk for heart disease and, possibly, cancer.
The risk of getting too much iron from foods is considered to
be quite low. However, the risks of long-term use of moderate-
to-high doses of iron, 25 to 75 mg. a day, are unknown.

MAGNESIUM

Q: What is magnesium?

A: Magnesium is a silvery-white metallic element related
to calcium and zinc. Because magnesium is very light
but strong, alloys of it are used in airplanes, parts of cars,
ladders, portable tools and luggage. Magnesium is also the
major mineral in asbestos and talcum powder. ''Milk of
magnesia'' is a poorly absorbed form of magnesium that
works by drawing water into the intestine.

Q: In what foods is magnesium found?

A: Whole grains, nuts, avocados, beans and dark green leafy vegetables are good sources. Food processing can result in great losses of magnesium. Little magnesium is left, for example, in white flour and rice, and practically none in sugar, alcohol, fats and oils.

Q: What role does magnesium play in the body?

A: Magnesium is necessary for every major biologic process in the body, including the production of energy from sugar and the manufacture of genetic material. It is important for muscle contraction, nerve conduction and blood-vessel tone. Magnesium interacts with calcium to regulate how much calcium enters cells to control such vital functions as heartbeat. Low intakes of magnesium have been associated with high blood pressure and heart disease.

Q: Has magnesium been used successfully to treat any diseases?

A: Yes. Intravenous magnesium, given during a heart attack, cuts in half a person's chances of developing arrhythmia, or irregular heartbeat, or of dying from heart stoppage, several studies have shown. The researchers for one of these studies say that intravenous magnesium "is simple, cheap and free of serious side effects" and works as well as drugs given to dissolve blood clots. In another study, people who received intravenous magnesium after heart bypass surgery were less likely to develop heartbeat problems and required less time on respiratory support than those not getting magnesium.

Chronic magnesium deficiency in animals has been shown to result in microscopic changes in the heart arteries, as well as in scarlike changes in the heart muscle itself—changes that were followed by calcium deposits that harden tissue and impair its ability to function normally.

Q: Has magnesium been used to treat any other problems?

A: In a recent study, supplementation with 4.5 grams of magnesium a day improved insulin response in the body, making it easier for older people to metabolize sugar, and so, maintain lower blood levels of both insulin and sugar. The researchers believe adequate amounts of magnesium allow insulin to move into cells easier, and so, improve the cells' ability to burn sugar for energy. Magnesium also apparently improves insulin secretion.

Q: You mentioned blood pressure. How is magnesium associated with that?

A: Several studies suggest that magnesium deficiency may contribute to high blood pressure. And magnesium supplements or intravenous magnesium therapy can lower blood pressure, by relaxing constricted blood vessels. In a Japanese study, when people with mild to moderately high blood pressure were given oral magnesium supplements for four weeks, their blood pressures dropped considerably. In another study, magnesium supplementation lowered blood pressure in people with diabetes.

Q: Is magnesium used to treat any other illnesses?

A: In one study, British researchers noted that people with chronic fatigue syndrome had abnormally low red-blood-cell magnesium levels. When 15 of these people were given injections of magnesium sulfate every week for six weeks, seven reported great improvement. And all but three reported some improvement in energy, less pain and less anxiety when compared with a similar group not receiving supplemental magnesium. Most researchers, however, believe further study is needed to see if the effect continues and to determine if oral magnesium might offer similar benefits.

Magnesium is important for normal bone structure, and in a small study, magnesium given along with calcium significantly increased bone-mineral density of postmenopausal women on estrogen therapy.

At least two studies indicate that intravenous magnesium relieves wheezing and improves lung function in people with asthma.

And in one study, oral magnesium treatment for two weeks prior to menstruation was found to relieve both premenstrual and menstrual symptoms, both physical and emotional.

Q: Do most people get enough magnesium in their diets?

A: No, they tend to fall somewhat short of RDA recommendations for this mineral. Studies indicate that someone eating about 2,000 calories a day would get about 240 mg. of magnesium. The RDA for adult men is 350 mg.; for women, it's 250 mg. A USDA study showed that the average daily intake for women was slightly more than 200 mg., and for men, close to 300 mg.

Q: What are signs of magnesium deficiency?

A: Symptoms of magnesium deficiency are slow to develop because of reserves in the body. They include nausea, muscle weakness, irritability, diarrhea, confusion, tremors, loss of coordination, muscle cramps, dizziness, apathy, depression and irregular heartbeat.

Q: Who is likely to be deficient in magnesium?

A: Marginal magnesium deficiency is now considered to be very common. In most people, magnesium deficiency is likely to be the result of malnutrition, diabetes, intestinal absorption problems, prolonged diarrhea and alcoholism. People taking diuretics or digitalis for long periods of time or on tube or intravenous feeding may also develop a deficiency. So do many pregnant women and people who exercise strenuously.

MAGNESIUM
QUICK-REFERENCE GUIDE

RDA
For men 350 mg.; for women, 250 mg.

SOURCES
Whole grains, nuts, avocados, beans and dark green leafy vegetables.

SIGNS OF DEFICIENCY
Loss of appetite, nausea, vomiting, diarrhea, confusion, tremors, loss of coordination, muscle cramps, dizziness, apathy, depression and irregular heartbeat.

POSSIBLE TOXICITY PROBLEMS
Magnesium has a good safety record. Symptoms of overdose have been seen with abuse of magnesium-containing antacids. They include low blood pressure, lethargy, weakness, slight slurring of speech, unsteadiness, fluid retention, and nausea and vomiting. The lowest level on record causing harm to an individual with healthy kidneys is 1,700 mg. a day. People with kidney problems should take supplemental magnesium only with medical supervision. Experts consider a safe dose for such people to be about 600 mg. a day.

POTASSIUM

Q: What is potassium?

A: Potassium is a soft, silvery-white metal found in nature only in compounds, called potassium salts. It is one of the most abundant minerals in the body. Unlike sodium, which is found mostly in the fluid outside of cells, potassium is located almost entirely within cells. It is concentrated chiefly in muscles, but it is also found in skin and other tissues. The body does not store potassium but must constantly replenish it through diet.

Q: In what foods is potassium found?

A: Fruits (including bananas) and vegetables and their juices are the best sources. Baked potatoes, yams, avocados, prunes, beet greens, carrot juice and raisins all offer good amounts of potassium, as do shellfish and beans.

Q: What role does potassium play in the body?

A: It plays a major role in many important functions, including muscle contraction, nerve conduction, regulation of heartbeat, energy production, and the manufacture of genetic material and protein.

Q: Has potassium deficiency been associated with any diseases?

A: In several population studies, a low intake of potassium seems to be linked with an increase in blood pressure and in death from stroke.

In one study, researchers reported they had induced blood pressure to rise an average of about six points in people with high blood pressure by restricting their potassium intake for 10 days.

And in a 12-year investigation of residents of a California community, men eating the least amount of potassium were nearly three times more likely to die of a stroke than those eating large amounts of potassium. For women in the low-intake group, the risk was about five times higher than women in the high-intake group. The difference between the two groups: about 665 mg. of potassium—just one serving of a potassium-rich vegetable, such as a large baked potato.

Q: Is an increased intake of potassium ever used to treat high blood pressure?

A: In several studies, increased dietary intake of potassium or potassium supplementation resulted in a modest decrease in blood pressure in people with high blood pressure.

One study, by researchers in Naples, Italy, recruited 54 men and women whose drug regimens kept their blood pressure below 160/95 mm Hg. For the next year, half the study participants sharply increased their intake of high-potassium foods without changing the total number of calories they consumed. The others maintained their normal eating habits. The doctors supervised the withdrawal of drugs from the people in both groups. At the end of the year, 81 percent of the people on the high-potassium diet were able to reduce their blood-pressure-drug use by over 50 percent. Only 29 percent of the "normal diet" group could cut back that far.

Q: What about stroke?

A: Increased potassium intake has not been studied for its ability to reduce the incidence of stroke, but some doctors do recommend increased potassium intake or potassium supplements to their patients with a strong family history of stroke.

Q: How is potassium thought to lower blood pressure?

A: Potassium interacts with sodium to regulate the body's fluid balance. Potassium enhances excretion of sodium through the urine, which leads to a decrease in blood volume, which in turn leads to a drop in blood pressure. Potassium depletion makes the body retain more fluid in response to a large dose of salt.

Q: Is potassium used to treat any other physical problems?

A: Potassium is added to sports drinks to replace the 700 to 800 mg. of potassium that can be lost in a few hours of heavy sweating. Although potassium depletion leads to muscle weakness and fatigue, extra potassium is not known to improve athletic performance in someone who is not deficient.

Q: How much potassium do people get in their diets?

A: Studies show that potassium intake varies widely. People who eat large amounts of fruits and vegetables may get up to 8 to 10 grams a day of potassium. Most people get about 2,500 mg. a day. African-Americans seem to have generally low intakes of 1,000 mg. or so a day.

People who follow the USDA recommendation to eat three vegetables and two fruits a day would get about 3,500 mg. of potassium a day. That falls right in the middle of potassium experts' recommendations to aim for 3,000 to 4,000 mg. a day—equivalent to eight bananas or 3½ baked potatoes.

Q: Who is at risk for potassium deficiency?

A: People who use potassium-depleting diuretics (blood-pressure-reducing drugs that work by increasing urine output) are at highest risk for deficiency. People who sweat a lot or who have chronic diarrhea are also at increased risk for deficiency.

Q: What are signs of potassium deficiency?

A: Symptoms of deficiency include easy fatigue, generalized weakness, muscle pains, abnormal heartbeat, drowsiness and irrational behavior.

POTASSIUM
QUICK-REFERENCE GUIDE

RDA
Since potassium is found in most foods and seldom is lacking in diets, there is no RDA for potassium. The National Research Council estimates the minimum requirement to be 1,600 to 2,000 milligrams a day.

SOURCES
Fruits (including bananas) and vegetables and their juices are the best sources. Baked potatoes, yams, avocados, prunes, beet greens, carrot juice and raisins all offer good amounts of potassium, as do shellfish and beans.

SIGNS OF DEFICIENCY
Fatigue, weakness, muscle pains, abnormal heartbeat, drowsiness and irrational behavior.

POSSIBLE TOXICITY PROBLEMS
High doses of several grams—the result of misuse of supplements or salt substitutes—can result in heart failure. Other symptoms of toxicity include muscle weakness, mental confusion, numbness and tingling of the extremities, and cold, pale skin. Potassium supplements containing more than 99 mg. per tablet are available only by prescription, and should be used only with medical supervision. Diabetics, people with kidney problems, people taking a potassium-sparing diuretic called spironolactone, and people taking ACE inhibitors may all retain potassium. Their use of potassium supplements should be medically supervised.

SELENIUM

Q: What is selenium?

A: Selenium is one of the trace minerals essential for human health. It is closely related chemically to sulfur, another essential nutrient, but is needed in much smaller amounts. In 1989, selenium was given an RDA of 70 mcg. for men and 55 mcg. for women, making it the most recent of the trace minerals to get an RDA.

Q: In what foods is selenium found?

A: The amount of selenium found in foods depends on how much selenium is in the soil in which the food is grown. In general, the best sources are broccoli, mushrooms, cabbage, celery, cucumbers, onions, garlic, radishes, brewer's yeast, grains, fish and organ meats.

Q: What role does selenium play in the body?

A: Like vitamins E and C, and beta-carotene, selenium acts as an antioxidant. It is essential for the formation of an enzyme, **glutathione peroxidase**, that is known to have powerful antioxidant properties. In studies, selenium appears to help prevent some types of cancer and heart disease, to boost the body's infection-fighting abilities, to detoxify potential cancer-causing heavy metals, such as mercury and cadmium, and to dampen inflammation, making it a potential help in the fight against chronic inflammatory diseases like rheumatoid arthritis.

Q: What can you tell me about selenium and cancer?

A: A number of studies now show that cancer rates go up when intakes of selenium go down. In fact, around the world, cancer rates follow the same lines as selenium-poor soil. Rapid City, South Dakota, for instance, an area of selenium-rich soil, has about half the cancer rate of the state of Ohio, an area with selenium-poor soil. In more than 20 countries, the findings are the same. The lower the selenium intake, the higher the incidence of leukemia and cancers of the colon, rectum, pancreas, breast, ovary, prostate, bladder, skin, and in men, lungs.

Blood samples taken of large groups of people show that people are more likely to develop cancer if they have low blood levels of selenium. In animal experiments, selenium supplementation significantly reduced the incidence of cancer of the liver, skin, breast and colon.

Q: And what about heart disease? How does selenium affect it?

A: Here again, as with vitamins E and C, selenium acts as an antioxidant to help prevent the buildup of artery-clogging fats and accompanying blood-vessel-wall damage. A number of studies also suggest that selenium, especially in combination with vitamin E, may protect against tissue damage related to restricted blood flow.

In addition to this, selenium, like vitamin E, has the ability to inhibit blood-cell clumping, also known as platelet aggregation.

Q: You said selenium boosts the body's infection-fighting abilities. How does it do that?

A: Exactly how selenium enhances immune function remains unclear. As with other antioxidants, however, it appears to help protect white blood cells from the free radicals they generate in the process of fighting infection.

For instance, selenium protects one type of white blood cell, macrophages, against the free radicals they generate when they engulf and destroy bacteria.

Q: How does selenium protect against heavy-metal poisoning?

A: Here again, the precise mechanism is not known, but it is thought to combine with the metal and become a harmless compound.

Q: You said selenium might help inflammatory conditions, such as arthritis. Any studies showing it does so?

A: Unfortunately, scientific documentation on its use for this and other conditions is mostly anecdotal. However, injectable and oral selenium/vitamin-E preparations are used, with reported good results, in veterinary practices to relieve arthritis inflammation in dogs and other animals.

Q: Do most people get enough selenium in their diets?

A: Dietary surveys indicate that most people get about the RDA of selenium. However, evidence seems to indicate that amounts larger than the RDA are required for protection against cancer and heart disease. For that reason, some researchers recommend supplementing your diet with 50 to 200 mcg. selenium a day.

Q: What are signs of deficiency?

A: In animals, a form of muscular dystrophy, with severe muscle wasting, develops as a sign of selenium deficiency. In humans, severe muscle pain and, eventually, an inability to walk were noted in one woman who developed selenium deficiency. In parts of China where deficiency results from selenium-poor soil, a form of heart disease develops. It includes heart enlargement, fast rhythm, abnormal electrocardiogram and, in severe cases, heart failure and death.

Q: Who's likely to be deficient in selenium?

A: Selenium deficiency is considered rare in the United States. The few reported cases have been in people on tube or intravenous feedings that did not supply adequate amounts of this nutrient.

SELENIUM
QUICK-REFERENCE GUIDE

RDA
For men, 70 mcg.; for women, 55 mcg.

SOURCES
Broccoli, mushrooms, cabbage, celery, cucumbers, onions, garlic, radishes, brewer's yeast, grains, fish and organ meats.

SIGNS OF DEFICIENCY
Muscle pain and wasting, heart problems.

POSSIBLE TOXICITY PROBLEMS
The level of dietary selenium that causes chronic poisoning is not known with certainty. However, 5 mg. a day from foods results in fingernail changes and hair loss. One man taking 1,000 mcg. a day for a year and a half developed damaged fingernails and garlic breath. The early signs of selenium toxicity include fatigue, irritability and dry hair. Workers, such as miners, exposed to high amounts of selenium develop garlic breath, dry skin and hair and brittle nails, nausea, vomiting and nervous-system problems, such as unusual or diminished sensations or paralysis.

ZINC

Q: What is zinc?

A: Zinc is a silvery-blue metal used to galvanize iron and as a component in flashlight batteries. It is essential for human health. About two grams of zinc are found in the body at any time.

Q: In what foods is zinc found?

A: Oysters, beef, pork and beef liver, lamb, crab, wheat germ and miso (fermented soybean paste) are all good sources of zinc.

Q: What role does zinc play in the body?

A: Zinc is known to be involved in the structure and function of cell membranes and in the production of more than 200 enzymes, including those involved in the production of nucleic acid, a cell's genetic material. And it's known to be essential for proper wound healing and healthy skin, for a strong immune system, for normal taste and smell and sexual function, for bone metabolism and for vision, among other things.

Q: So it's involved in many functions. What would you say are its most important functions?

A: Certainly one that has garnered a lot of study recently is zinc's role in the immune system.

Q: What about it?

A: Zinc is considered one of the most important of the many nutrients needed for proper immune function. People who are zinc deficient are much more likely to develop infections, and many researchers believe the decline in immune function in older people is due, at least in part, to deficiencies of zinc and other nutrients important for proper immunity. In one study, zinc supplementation (220 mg. twice a day for one month) increased the number of infection-fighting white blood cells in healthy people older than age 70. There was no such improvement in a group that received no supplementation.

Another study also suggests that one form of zinc, called zinc gluconate, can help to reduce symptoms of the common cold. Student volunteers who took 184 mg. a day of zinc gluconate as lozenges got over their colds in about four days of treatment, while students taking placebo lozenges were sick for an average of nine days. Zinc seems to work against colds only when it dissolves in the mouth, researchers point out. High zinc levels in saliva apparently affect facial nerve endings, drying up your runny nose and preventing the cold virus from multiplying.

Blood levels of zinc have been found to be low in people with AIDS, and researchers are currently looking at whether zinc supplementation can help maintain their immunity.

Q: You said zinc is essential for our ability to taste and smell. Does that mean we lose these senses if we're low on zinc?

A: Yes. People who are zinc deficient often have a poor sense of taste and smell. That can create a vicious circle. The loss of taste and smell often leads to poor appetite, which in turn leads to poor nourishment.

In fact, some researchers believe that anorexia nervosa, a condition characterized by loss of appetite and compulsive dieting, may be aggravated when initial dieting leads to zinc deficiency. And one study found that increasing the calorie intake of women suffering from anorexia nervosa—including providing them with a balanced diet that includes the RDA of zinc—initially lowered their blood zinc levels.

The researchers believe that's because the RDA of zinc (12 mg. for women) did not provide all the zinc needed for the tissue-building that accompanied the weight gain. It took upwards of 75 mg. of zinc supplementation, along with additional calories, for zinc blood levels to rise to normal in these women.

Q: And what about vision? Can zinc deficiency lead to loss of eyesight?

A: Zinc is involved in normal functions of the retina (the back of the eye). Degeneration of the central part of the retina, called macular degeneration, is a leading cause of visual loss in the elderly. In one study, healthy older people given 100 mg. of zinc, twice a day, for one to two years had significantly less vision loss from macular degeneration than a similar group that got placebos.

Q: Does zinc play a role in cancer prevention?

A: Findings are contradictory. Some studies indicate that adequate zinc intake protects against the development of cancer. In others, however, zinc-deficient animals actually had slower tumor growth than those with adequate intakes. Zinc may help to protect against cancer by helping neutralize certain cancer-causing agents, such as cadmium, a heavy metal, and by keeping the immune system at optimum operating capacity. On the other hand, since zinc is necessary for normal cell growth, a deficiency might also impair the growth of established cancer cells.

Since zinc deficiency leads to serious symptoms, however, induced zinc deficiency would never be used to treat cancer. For established cancer (in animals), this treatment has too many adverse side effects to be used for humans. Same with some other minerals, too.

Q: What does zinc have to do with sexual function?

A: In men, zinc deficiency leads to a reduction in the production of testosterone, the main male hormone that stimulates the development of male reproductive organs, including the prostate, and the secondary sex characteristics, such as facial hair and muscles. Men with fertility problems who also have low blood levels of zinc often benefit from a course of zinc supplementation. Zinc deficiency also leads to reduced sex drive. Adolescent boys who are low in zinc often have delayed puberty.

Q: Isn't zinc sometimes used to treat prostate problems?

A: It has been used to treat a kind of soft prostate enlargement called benign prostatic hyperplasia. And although there is some anecdotal evidence that about 80 mg. a day of zinc sulfate does help some men with this condition, there are no scientific studies to prove that it does, in fact, work.

Q: Anything else zinc is good for?

A: Zinc, like iron and other trace minerals, apparently plays a role in the body's production of neurotransmitters—brain chemicals that relay messages. In a study of people with head injuries, those who got about five times the amount of zinc normally found in intravenous formulas had significantly higher neurological scores, as assessed by a neurologist, a month after their accidents.

Topical zinc paste has been used to treat leg sores associated with poor circulation, and seems to make topical antibiotics work better against acne.

Q: Do people get enough zinc in their diets?

A: Apparently most people don't do too badly. A typical American diet furnishes 10 to 15 mg. of zinc a day, close to the RDA of 15 mg. for men, and 12 mg. for women. However, studies show that some groups of people are low on zinc.

Q: Who is at risk for zinc deficiency?

A: The elderly, people on reduced-calorie diets, and vegetarians (since zinc is found mostly in meats). Certain drugs, such as diuretics, and diseases (diabetes and alcoholism, for example) lead to increased zinc excretion and thus to a need for increased zinc intake. Excessive sweating can also cause significant zinc loss.

Q: What are signs of zinc deficiency?

A: Growth retardation, poor appetite, underfunctioning sex glands, mental lethargy, delayed wound healing, abnormalities of taste, smell and vision, skin changes and increased susceptibility to infection.

ZINC
QUICK-REFERENCE GUIDE

RDA
For men, 15 mg.; for women, 12 mg.

SOURCES
Good sources include oysters, beef, pork and beef liver, lamb, crab, wheat germ and miso (fermented soybean paste).

SIGNS OF DEFICIENCY
Growth retardation, poor appetite, underfunctioning sex glands, mental lethargy, delayed wound healing, abnormalities of taste, smell and vision, skin changes and increased susceptibility to infection.

POSSIBLE TOXICITY PROBLEMS
Zinc competes with copper for intestinal absorption; some researchers believe that people taking amounts of zinc as low as 15 mg. should also be getting about 2 mg. of copper.
   In a recent study, high doses of zinc depressed immune function. Even 25 mg. of zinc, considered a fairly low dose, led to poorer immune function after six months of supplementation.

CHLORIDE, FLUORIDE, MANGANESE, MOLYBDENUM, PHOSPHORUS, SODIUM

Chloride

Q: What is chloride?

A: Chloride, a common water purifier and bleach, is an essential nutrient for humans. Its name is from the Greek, meaning "greenish-yellow." Only water-soluble chloride compounds exist in nature. Chloride gas, which can be created in the laboratory, is a very toxic substance used in chemical warfare.

Q: What role does chloride play in the body?

A: Chloride ions act as **electrolytes**—they are part of the mineral-laden fluid found both inside and outside the body's cells. This fluid conveys electrical charges throughout the body and helps move molecules in and out of cells. It is known to help to activate nerve impulses.

Chloride is most abundant in the fluid outside of cells, but some is also found in cells. Chloride is also concentrated in the stomach's food-dissolving acids, and in the fluid found around the brain and spine.

Q: I've never known of anyone being low in this nutrient. Does that ever happen?

A: Only rarely. The same sorts of things that cause sodium loss—heavy sweating, prolonged vomiting and diarrhea—can cause chloride loss. Table salt, which is sodium chloride, corrects both deficiencies.

Q: How much chloride are people supposed to get?

A: The suggested range for adults is 1,700 to 5,100 mg. a day. Most adults average 3,500 to 7,000 mg. a day, due to the typical American diet, which is high in salt.

Q: What are symptoms of chloride deficiency?

A: In a case where an infant formula was inadvertently made without chloride, the infants failed to gain weight and suffered from constipation, too-alkaline blood and electrolyte abnormalities. When chloride was added, the infants promptly improved.

Fluoride

Q: What is fluoride?

A: Fluoride is a nonmetallic compound that is also toxic as a gas. Fluoride is known to be beneficial to humans, specifically for its role in maintaining bones and tooth enamel, but it has not yet been proven to be essential for human health.

Q: I know that fluoride is often added to some brands of toothpaste, and even to some municipal water systems to help reduce cavities. Does it really work for that?

A: Yes, when adequate amounts of fluoride are incorporated into tooth enamel, the rate of tooth decay is reduced by 25 percent, or even further. Studies show that it works not only for children's teeth, but for adults, too. In one study of adults older than 54, a group using fluoridated toothpaste for a year had 41 percent less tooth decay and 67 percent less root decay than a group using a nonfluoridated toothpaste. More than half of people age 65 or older have root decay, largely because gum lines recede with age.

Q: Then why do some people get so upset over the fluoridation of water?

A: For several reasons. Some apparently believe people can get all the fluoride they need from toothpaste or mouthwash. And some believe, perhaps with good reason, that not all of fluoride's possible long-term risks are known. A recent study, for instance, suggests that sodium fluoride, the compound that is usually added to water supplies, enhances the body's uptake of aluminum, a metal that some researchers believe may be linked with the development of Alzheimer's disease.

Q: Are there any problems associated with fluoride toxicity?

A: Chronic fluoride toxicity is known to cause abnormal hardening of the bones and is associated with joint pain and stiffness, weakness and occasionally nerve damage and paralysis. This condition occurs only after years of daily exposures to 20 to 80 mg. of fluoride, far in excess of the average individual's intake in the United States.

And fluoride can be toxic. Consuming 2.5 to 5 grams at one time can be fatal to adults and children. In children, amounts of more than 2.5 mg. a day can lead to mottled tooth enamel.

Q: Someone told me fluoride may cause cancer. Is that true?

A: No one knows for sure. A report filed in February 1991 by a committee convened by the U.S. National Toxicology Program to clear up the fluoride question, found "equivocal" evidence linking fluoride to cancer. Some experts say that studies examining fluoride's potential cancer risk show that risk is small. Others say the results provide clear evidence that fluoride causes cancer. One researcher, in a controversial study released in 1977, found people living in the nation's 10 largest cities with fluoridated water suffered 15 percent more cancer than those living in the 10 largest cities with no fluoride in the water. Other experts contend that exposure to fluoride may set the state for multiple chemical sensitivities. However, there is little research to support this claim.

Q: You said fluoride is involved in bone health. Is it ever used to treat bone diseases such as osteoporosis?

A: Yes, sodium fluoride has been used experimentally, along with calcium, to promote the growth of new bone in people with osteoporosis. In fact, it does promote new bone growth, but some researchers worry that the new bone growth is too brittle to bear weight, and there is some research to support that concern. In a study of three groups of postmenopausal women from three different communities with different levels of fluoride in the water, the group with the highest water levels of fluoride had double the incidence of bone fractures compared with the low-fluoride group. These researchers point out that fluoride probably is helpful for bones and teeth in small amounts, but in larger amounts becomes counterproductive.

Q: Is fluoride good for anything else?

A: Researchers have noted that people drinking fluoride-rich water have a lower incidence of soft-tissue calcification, a problem we talked about in the section on vitamin D. That means calcium is less likely to end up in their arteries, heart valves, tendons and other tissues, where it can harden tissues and make them malfunction.

Q: How much fluoride are people supposed to get?

A: There is no RDA for fluoride. The recommended range is 1.5 to 4 mg. a day. In the United States, most people are somewhere in that range, depending mostly on whether their drinking water contains fluoride.

Q: Do any foods contain fluoride?

A: Yes, tea is a rich source of fluoride. One cup of brewed black tea contains from 1 to 4 mg. Seafood is also a good source.

Manganese

Q: What is manganese?

A: Manganese is a white, powdery mineral, essential for human health. It is sometimes confused with magnesium, which looks similar but has different properties.

Q: What role does manganese play in the body?

A: Researchers know that manganese's major role is as an antioxidant. It is involved in chemical reactions involving energy production, nerve-cell metabolism, muscle contraction and bone growth. Details of its role in the body, however, are mostly unknown.

Manganese-deficiency states have been induced in animals —they include defective growth and neurologic disorders— but manganese deficiency is unknown in humans. Only one incident of what might have been a manganese deficiency has been reported, in a man who lived for four months on a manganese-deficient diet. His symptoms included impaired blood clotting, reddening of his black hair and beard, slowed growth of hair and nails, and scaly skin.

Q: So people are never deficient in manganese?

A: Apparently not.

Q: Is manganese ever toxic?

A: Yes, exposure to large amounts of manganese, such as is found in Peruvian manganese miners, can cause "manganese madness," a condition marked first by unaccountable laughter, heightened sexual response, impulsiveness, inability to fall asleep, delusions and hallucinations. This state is followed by depression, and finally, by symptoms similar to that of Parkinson's disease—slow, sparse movements, muscular rigidity, tremor and balance problems.

Q: Is there a recommended daily amount?

A: Yes, 2.5 to 5 mg. a day is considered a safe and adequate amount. And dietary studies show that intakes well above that amount are still within a safe range.

Q: In what foods is manganese found?

A: Many foods contain this mineral. Nuts, vegetables and fruits are especially good sources.

Molybdenum

Q: What is molybdenum?

A: Molybdenum is a essential trace mineral, known to play a role in the production of several enzymes.

Q: What role does molybdenum play in the body?

A: One of its roles is to help the body to detoxify sulfites, sulfur compounds added to foods as preservatives and also created in the body as a result of protein metabolism. Molybdenum may also act as an antioxidant, since, in China, deficiencies have been associated with a large increase in

throat cancer. However, there is no scientific evidence that
supplemental molybdenum protects against cancer.

Q: In what foods is molybdenum found?

A: Not all foods have been assessed for their molybdenum content, but in one survey, the foods most
likely to contain this mineral were milk, beans, breads
and cereals.

Q: How much molybdenum do most people get?

A: One study found ranges from 76 to 109 mcg. a day,
within the suggested range of 75 to 250 mcg. a day.

Q: Does molybdenum deficiency ever occur?

A: Rarely. Even in laboratory animals, it is hard to cause
a deficiency. Only in people on long-term tube or
intravenous feeding or with rare genetic inability to utilize
molybdenum has a deficiency been seen.

Q: What are signs of molybdenum deficiency?

A: In one man who apparently developed such a deficiency as a result of improper tube feeding, symptoms
included rapid rates of heartbeat and breathing, headache,
night blindness, mental disturbances, irritability, nausea and
vomiting. Eventually, disorientation, fluid retention and coma
resulted. This man also had biochemical signs of problems
metabolizing sulfites and purines, components of proteins.
Since researchers at that time knew that molybdenum was

necessary for the metabolism of both of these compounds, they tried giving the man molybdenum. That resulted in a reversal of his symptoms.

Q: Is this stuff ever toxic?

A: Yes. Dietary intake of 10 to 15 mg. has been associated with symptoms similar to gout—increased blood levels of uric acid and swelling in the joints, especially the big toe. Molybdenum also interferes with copper absorption. Amounts of 500 mcg. a day have been found to cause significant body losses of copper.

Phosphorus

Q: What is phosphorus?

A: Phosphorus is a nonmetallic element that in its unnatural free form glows in the dark and breaks into fire spontaneously upon exposure to air. It exists in nature only in combined forms, usually with calcium. Phosphorus is used to make matches, detergents and fertilizers. It is also used as a food preservative.

Q: In what foods is phosphorus found?

A: Meats, fish and poultry, eggs, cheese and milk, nuts, beans and grains are the best sources. Fruits and vegetables, especially dark green leafy vegetables, also contribute some phosphorus to the diet.

Q: What role does phosphorus play in the body?

A: Phosphorus is considered an important nutrient. It takes part in almost every metabolic reaction in the body. It also interacts with calcium to mineralize bones and teeth. It is an essential element of a cell's genetic material and of blood fats and cell membranes. It is also important in the normal transmission of nerve impulses.

Q: What are signs of deficiency?

A: Reduced bone mineralization, loss of appetite, weakness, muscle tremors and bone pain are the most common symptoms.

Q: Who's likely to be deficient?

A: In the United States, phosphorus deficiency is considered rare because phosphorus is found in many different foods. It is possible to become deficient in this mineral, though, if you are taking large amounts of aluminum-containing antacids, which block the intestinal absorption of phosphorus. Persistent vomiting, disorders of vitamin D metabolism, kidney or liver disorders, or alcoholism can also cause phosphorus deficiencies. Up to 20 percent of all hospitalized people have been identified as having low levels of phosphorus in the blood.

Q: What is the RDA for phosphorus?

A: The RDA is the same as for calcium—800 mg. a day.

Sodium

Q: What is sodium?

A: Sodium is a soft, silvery-white metal. It is usually found as one of a number of compounds, of which sodium chloride, or table salt, is the most familiar. Salt was probably the first food additive and preservative to be used. In ancient times, salt was considered so important that it was often used as a form of money. In fact, the word "salary" comes from the use of salt as a form of payment to Roman soldiers.

Q: I thought sodium *was* salt. Isn't that the case?

A: No. Sodium is an element, while common salt is a compound containing both sodium and chloride. Salt is about 40 percent sodium.

Q: In what foods is sodium found?

A: Nearly all foods contain some sodium. Processed foods such as frozen dinners, lunch meats and snacks (pretzels and potato chips, for example) contain large amounts, as do cheese and shellfish.

Q: What role does sodium play in the body?

A: Sodium is an electrolyte. It is important for maintaining the body's fluid balance and for moving fluids in and out of cells. It is also important in the transmission of nerve impulses, in heart function, and in protein and carbohydrate metabolism.

Q: Do doctors still recommend I reduce my salt intake to lower my blood pressure?

A: Yes. A high-salt diet has been associated with increased risk for high blood pressure. But researchers now know that intake of potassium, calcium and magnesium also influence blood pressure. A proper balance of all four of these minerals is important for normal blood pressure and heartbeat.

Q: What are signs of sodium deficiency?

A: Symptoms include loss of appetite, loss of thirst, severe muscle cramps and weakness, vomiting and irritability. A severe deficiency results in death.

Q: Who's likely to be deficient?

A: In most countries, sodium deficiency is considered unusual. However, people suffering from prolonged diarrhea, kidney disease, or who sweat heavily due to strenuous activity in hot climates may develop sodium deficiency.

Q: What is the RDA for sodium?

A: Because deficiency is so rare, there is no RDA for sodium. An amount of about 500 mg. a day is considered safe and adequate. Most people eat three or four grams of sodium a day.

INFORMATIONAL AND MUTUAL-AID GROUPS

American College of Nutrition
722 Robert E. Lee Dr.
Wilmington, NC 28412
(919) 452-1222

A membership organization for clinicians and researchers in the field of nutrition. Publishes Journal of the American College of Nutrition. *Can verify if a doctor is a member of this organization.*

American Dietetic Association
430 N. Michigan Ave.
Chicago, IL 60611

For a list of registered dietitians in your area, send your request, along with a self-addressed stamped envelope and $1.

American Holistic Medical Association
2002 Eastlake Ave. East
Seattle, WA 98102
(206) 322-6842

Can refer you to a doctor in your area who is a member of this organization.

American Society for Clinical Nutrition
9650 Rockville Pike
Bethesda, MD 20814
(301) 530-7110

A membership organization for clinicians and researchers engaged in nutrition research. Publishes American Journal of Clinical Nutrition. *Can verify if a doctor is a member of this organization.*

Society for Nutrition Education
2001 Killebrew Dr.
Suite 340
Minneapolis, MN 55425-1882
(612) 854-0035
(800) 235-6690

Membership organization for nutrition educators from the fields of dietetics, public health, home economics, medicine, industry and education. Sells nutrition education materials and films. Publishes Journal of Nutrition Education.

GLOSSARY

Adrenal glands: Small endocrine glands; one is located on each kidney. The glands secrete a number of hormones, including epinephrine (sometimes called adrenaline), the stimulating hormone that makes our hearts race and palms sweat when we are frightened. The adrenal glands also secrete more than 30 steroid hormones, which are involved in many functions, including muscle building, sex drive and the reduction of inflammation.

Allopathic: Pertaining to allopathy, the form of medicine practiced by M.D.'s.

Amino acids: Compounds that form the chief constituents of protein. Twenty amino acids are necessary for the body to make protein, a process called protein synthesis.

Antioxidant: A molecule that helps limit potentially harmful oxidative reactions by neutralizing free radicals. Free radicals are molecular fragments that attempt to steal electrons from other molecules. An antioxidant donates an electron to the free radical, thereby neutralizing it. Nutrients that act as antioxidants include vitamins C and E, beta-carotene and selenium.

Ascorbate: See **Vitamin C**.

Ascorbic acid: See **Vitamin C**.

B complex: The members of the B vitamin family, including biotin, B6, B12, folic acid, niacin, pantothenic acid, riboflavin and thiamin.

Beriberi: A thiamin-deficiency disease, with symptoms including mental confusion, loss of appetite, muscular weakness, trouble walking, paralysis of the limbs and eye problems.

Beta-carotene: The orange pigment found in carrots, sweet potatoes and many other fruits and vegetables that can be converted in the body into vitamin A. Beta-carotene is an antioxidant, a function independent of its conversion to vitamin A.

Bioavailability: The degree to which a nutrient or other substance becomes available for use in the body after ingestion or injection.

Bioflavonoids: Substances often found in fruits containing vitamin C that are occasionally considered to be essential vitamins for humans. Their vitamin status, however, has not been established.

Biotin: A member of the vitamin B complex.

Brewer's yeast: The same bitter-tasting yeast that is used to brew beer, and a rich source of a variety of nutrients, including thiamin, riboflavin, niacin, B_6, pantothenic acid, biotin, folic acid, chromium, selenium and other trace minerals.

Calcitriol: A hormone and the biologically active form of vitamin D.

Calcium: The most abundant mineral in the body, necessary for hard bones and teeth and for proper muscle and nerve function. Dissolved calcium is an essential part of the fluid that surrounds cells.

Carbohydrate: A compound of carbon, hydrogen and oxygen. One of three classes of nutrients in food that provide energy to the body. (Fats and sugars are the other two classes.) Examples of carbohydrates include grains and pasta.

Carotenoids: Any of a group of red, yellow or orange pigments that are found in foods such as carrots, sweet potatoes and leafy green vegetables. The body converts these substances to vitamin A.

Catechin: A type of bioflavonoid, found in fruits that contain vitamin C and not considered an essential nutrient.

Celiac disease: A problem of intestinal absorption, usually diagnosed in early adulthood, related to a sensitivity to gluten (a protein in wheat). Symptoms include large, bulky, frothy, foul-smelling, pale-colored stools containing much fat. Recurrent attacks of diarrhea and stomach cramps, weight loss and malnutrition also occur with this disease.

Cervical dysplasia: Possibly precancerous changes in the cells lining the surface of the cervix—the neck of the uterus. Cervical dysplasia is usually discovered as a result of a Pap smear.

Chlorine: An essential nutrient, usually gotten as table salt (sodium chloride).

Choline: A nutrient, once considered a B vitamin, whose vitamin status has not been established. Involved in the production of certain neurotransmitters.

Chromium: An essential trace element, which the body needs to be able to burn sugar for energy.

Cobalamin: See **Vitamin B_{12}**.

Coenzymes: Substances that are vital participants in many of the chemical reactions that take place in our bodies. Vitamins and minerals are coenzymes for all chemical reactions in the body.

Collagen: Connective tissue, found throughout the body, which helps to maintain the structure of tissues, including skin, muscles, gums, blood vessels and bone.

Copper: An essential trace mineral, necessary for the production of collagen and involved in the body's production of anti-inflammatory enzymes.

Crohn's disease: An inflammation of the lower part of the small intestine. Symptoms, similar to inflammatory bowel disease, include bouts of diarrhea, cramping and fever. Causes absorption problems that can lead to malnutrition.

Daily Value (DV): A new term, coined by the U.S. Food and Drug Administration, designed to replace RDA, or Recommended Dietary Allowance. Daily Values will soon be appearing on food labels.

Deficiency-related disease: Any kind of condition or disease associated with low intake of a vitamin or mineral. Scurvy, for instance, is a vitamin C deficiency-related disease.

Dietitian: A health-care professional who provides dietary analysis and advice on improving eating habits.

Electrolyte: A substance that dissociates into ions (negatively or positively charged particles) when fused or in solution, and thus becomes capable of conducting electricity. In the body, major electrolytes are sodium, calcium, potassium, magnesium and chloride.

Element: A simple substance that cannot be decomposed by chemical means and which is made up of atoms that are alike in their chemical properties. See also **Trace Element**.

Enriched: A term used to denote a food in which vitamins and minerals lost during processing have been replaced. White enriched rice, for instance, contains some of the B vitamins lost when the rice is polished.

Estimated Safe and Adequate Daily Dietary Intake (ESADDI): A range of intake that may be given to a nutrient that does not have an RDA. Biotin, pantothenic acid, copper, fluoride, chromium and molybdenum all have ESADDIs rather than RDAs.

Fatty acid: An organic compound of carbon, hydrogen and oxygen that combines with glycerol to form fat. Fatty acids that are necessary for health are called essential fatty acids.

Folic acid: A B vitamin. A woman whose diet is low in folic acid at the time of conception has an increased risk of giving birth to a child with serious birth defects.

204 VITAMINS AND MINERALS

Food diary: A written record of the foods a person has eaten over a period of time, used to compile a nutritional analysis.

Fortified: A term used to denote a food to which has been added extra vitamins and minerals. Orange juice to which calcium has been added is considered a fortified food.

Glucose: Also known as dextrose. The type of sugar found in the blood and also found in some foods.

Glucose tolerance factor: An organic form of chromium, found in brewer's yeast, that enhances the body's response to insulin, helping it move glucose (sugar) into cells where it can be burned for energy. Glucose tolerance factor also includes niacin.

Glutathione peroxidase: An antioxidant enzyme, formed in the body, that requires the trace mineral selenium.

Goiter: Enlargement of the thyroid gland due to iodine deficiency.

HDL (High-density lipoprotein): A portion of cholesterol believed to transport cholesterol away from the tissues and to the liver, where it can be excreted.

Hemochromatosis: A genetic disorder in which there are excessive deposits of iron in the liver, heart, pancreas, skin and other organs, all of which are subject to serious damage from toxic free-radicals generated by the iron.

Hemoglobin: An oxygen-carrying iron-dependent protein found in red blood cells. Hemoglobin is low in some sorts of anemia.

Hesperidin: A type of bioflavonoid, found in fruits that contain vitamin C, and not considered an essential nutrient.

Homeopathy: A branch of medicine that believes that "like cures like" and that medicines that cause symptoms of diseases in healthy people will bring about cures in sick people.

Hyperthyroidism: Overactivity of the thyroid gland, characterized by headache, irritability, trembling, rapid pulse and insomnia.

Inositol: A sugar alcohol, sometimes found in multivitamin preparations, that is not considered essential for human health.

Insulin: A hormone secreted in response to blood sugar (glucose) that helps to transport glucose into cells and to store glucose in the liver and muscles.

Internist: A doctor who specializes in internal medicine—the diagnosis and treatment of diseases of the gastrointestinal tract, heart, kidney, liver and endocrine system.

Intrinsic factor: A protein that escorts B_{12} through the bowel and into the bloodstream.

Iodine: An essential nutrient, necessary for the body's production of thyroid hormones.

Iron: An essential trace mineral necessary for oxygen transportation throughout the body.

Isotretinoin: A synthetic vitamin-A-like substance used to treat severe acne; brand-name Accutane.

Jaundice: A yellowing of the eyes and skin caused by the buildup of yellow-colored bile pigments secreted by the liver. A sign of liver or gallbladder problems.

LDL (Low-density lipoprotein): The main portion of harmful cholesterol in the blood.

Macrocytic anemia: A type of anemia caused by folic-acid deficiency.

Magnesium: An essential mineral used in more than 300 biochemical reactions in the body.

Manganese: An essential trace mineral important for normal functioning of the brain and for bone structure.

Metabolism: The sum of the physical and chemical processes by which living organized substance is built up and maintained, and by which large molecules are broken down into smaller molecules to make energy available to the organism. In nutrition, metabolism usually refers to a complex chemical process, involving oxygen, that involves the release of energy from food. The metabolic process allows our bodies to convert the calories we take in as carbohydrates into usable energy.

Microflora: See **Microorganism.**

Microorganism: Microscopic organism, including bacteria living in the digestive tract. Also called **Microflora.**

Mineral: A nonorganic compound, one that does not contain carbon and does not originate from living organisms.

Molybdenum: An essential trace mineral that may act as an antioxidant.

Naturopathy: A healing art that emphasizes the body's natural healing forces. It is a drugless therapy that makes use of massage, light, heat, air and water.

Neural-tube defects: Serious birth defects associated with folic acid deficiency around the time of conception. These defects include failure of the fetal brain to develop or failure of the spinal cord to close.

Neurotransmitters: Chemical substances produced in the brain and nerves throughout the body that allow us to think, feel and otherwise function.

Niacin: A B vitamin essential for the metabolism of carbohydrates.

Niacinamide: A form of niacin, also known as nicotinamide.

Nicotinamide: A form of niacin, one of the B vitamins.

Nicotinic acid: A form of niacin, one of the B vitamins.

Nucleic acids: Extremely complex compounds that form the genetic material in cells and direct the synthesis of protein within the cell.

Nutrient: A biochemical substance used by the body that must be supplied in adequate amounts from foods consumed. There are six classes of nutrients: water, proteins, carbohydrates, fats, minerals and vitamins.

Nutritionist: An individual who provides information on food and nutrition. There is no accreditation process for nutritionists.

Osteomalacia: The adult equivalent of rickets, characterized by soft bones. Symptoms include bone pain and tenderness, and muscle weakness.

Osteopath: A doctor of osteopathy, a branch of medicine that is similar to traditional medicine but includes spinal manipulation and hands-on diagnosis and treatment.

Osteoporosis: Literally, porous bones. A condition most likely to occur in postmenopausal women.

Oxidation: A chemical process where a molecule combines with oxygen and loses electrons. Antioxidant nutrients such as vitamins C and E help control oxidation.

PABA: See **Para-aminobenzoic acid**.

Pantothenic acid: A B vitamin that plays a number of essential metabolic roles.

Para-aminobenzoic acid (PABA): A substance sometimes found in multivitamins but not considered to be essential for human health.

Pellagra: The classic niacin-deficiency disease, characterized by a reddish skin rash, especially on the face, hands and feet when they are exposed to sunlight, which later makes the skin rough and dark. The word means "rough skin" in Italian.

Peripheral: Outside the central region.

Pernicious anemia: A potentially fatal form of anemia caused by vitamin B_{12} deficiency, due to lack of gastric secretion of intrinsic factor, a protein that escorts B_{12} through the bowel into the bloodstream.

Phosphorus: An essential mineral that takes part in almost every metabolic reaction in the body.

Phylloquinone: The natural form of vitamin K.

Platelet aggregation: The clumping or sticking together of red blood cells, which can form blood clots in the vessels. Both vitamin E and selenium help reduce platelet aggregation.

Potassium: An essential mineral that may help protect against high blood pressure and stroke.

Provitamin: A vitamin precursor. A substance from which a vitamin can be made in the body.

Precursor: A substance from which a vitamin can be made in the body. Beta-carotene is a precursor for vitamin A.

Quasi-vitamins: Substances that are sometimes included in multivitamin formulas or that may be necessary nutrients for animals, but whose vitamin status for humans has not been established.

Quercetin: A type of bioflavonoid, found in fruits that contain vitamin C and not considered an essential nutrient.

Recommended Dietary Allowance (RDA): The levels of intake of essential nutrients that, on the basis of scientific knowledge, are judged by the Food and Nutrition Board of the National Academy of Sciences to be adequate to meet the known nutrient needs of practically all healthy persons.

Reference Daily Intake (RDI): A new term intended to replace the U.S.RDAs. RDIs are an average of the RDAs for all different age-groups.

Retinol: Preformed vitamin A.

Retinol equivalents (RE): Units of measure that make it possible to compare and convert the various forms of vitamin A, including preformed vitamin A, beta-carotene and other carotenoids, since all the different forms have different bioactivity in the body. One retinol equivalent equals 1 microgram of retinol or six micrograms of beta-carotene.

Riboflavin: Also called vitamin B_2, a nutrient necessary for energy metabolism and proper development of nerves and blood cells, for iron metabolism and adrenal gland function, for the formation of connective tissues, and for proper immune function.

Rickets: A vitamin D-deficiency disease characterized by bones so soft they bend under the body's weight.

Rutin: A type of bioflavonoid, found in fruits that contain vitamin C and not considered an essential nutrient.

Scurvy: A vitamin C-deficiency disease characterized by bleeding gums, pink or red hemorrhagic spots under the skin, rough skin, joint pain, fatigue, tissue degeneration and increased incidence of infection.

Selenium: A trace mineral that acts as an antioxidant and is thought to help protect against cancer and heart disease and to boost immunity.

Sensory neuropathy: Loss of the sense of touch and temperature variations in the hands or feet due to deterioration of the nerves that transmit these sensations.

Sodium: An essential nutrient involved in the conduction of electrical charges throughout the body, and essential for fluid balance.

Sugar: A sweet crystallizable material that is nutritionally important as a source of dietary carbohydrate and as a sweetener and preservative of other foods.

Sulfur: A tasteless, odorless chemical element that is used to make sulfuric acid and used commercially in many industrial processes.

Synthesis: Creation of a compound by union of elements composing it, done artificially or as a result of natural processes.

Synthesize: To produce by synthesis.

Synthetic: Produced by synthesis.

Thiamin: Also called vitamin B₁, a nutrient essential for energy metabolism and for nearly every cellular reaction taking place in the body—for normal development, growth, reproduction, maximum physical fitness and good health.

Tocopherol equivalents (TE): Units of measure that provide a basis that makes it possible to compare and convert the various forms of vitamin E, all of which have different levels of biological activity in the body. One tocopherol equivalent equals one milligram of d-alpha-tocopherol.

Trace element: See **Trace mineral**.

Trace mineral: A mineral essential to human health that is needed in amounts of less than 100 milligrams a day.

Triglycerides: Fatty acids, found in the blood, that at high levels contribute to the formation of heart disease.

Ultra-trace minerals: Minerals that are essential only in micrograms.

U.S.RDA: A term developed by the U.S. Food and Drug Administration that takes the highest RDAs—those for teenage boys—and applies them to the general population, regardless of age or gender.

Vitamin: An organic (carbon-containing) component of food found to be essential in small quantities for normal human metabolism, growth and physical well-being.

Vitamin A: A fat-soluble vitamin that is essential for, among other things, vision, strong immunity and proper cell development and maturation.

Vitamin B_1: See **Thiamin**.

Vitamin B_2: See **Riboflavin**.

Vitamin B_6: A B vitamin, also called pyridoxine, required for the proper functioning of more than 60 enzymes in the body, including those necessary for the body's metabolism of proteins, fats and carbohydrates.

Vitamin B_{12}: Also known as cobalamin. One of the B vitamins, with a molecule of cobalt at its center, essential for the normal functioning of all body cells, particularly those of the bone marrow, the nervous system and the gastrointestinal tract.

Vitamin C: Also known as ascorbate or ascorbic acid, it's a water-soluble vitamin with strong antioxidant properties. Helps to protect against cancer and heart disease, boosts immune function, speeds wound healing and provides various other benefits.

Vitamin D: A fat-soluble vitamin essential for the body's absorption of calcium.

Vitamin E: A fat-soluble vitamin whose main role in the body is to act as an antioxidant. Vitamin E helps to protect against heart disease and cancer.

Vitamin K: A fat-soluble vitamin essential for the clotting of blood.

Zinc: An essential trace mineral known to be involved in the structure and function of cell membranes and in the production of more than 200 enzymes, including those involved in the production of nucleic acid, a cell's genetic material. Zinc is essential for proper wound healing and healthy skin, strong immunity, normal taste and smell and sexual function, bone metabolism and vision, among other things.

SUGGESTED READING

Balch, James F., M.D., and Phyllis A. Balch. *Prescription for Nutritional Healing.* Garden City Park, N.Y.: Avery Publishing Group, 1990.

> *Organized A-to-Z by illness, a reference to using vitamins and minerals, herbs and nutritional supplements to treat numerous conditions.*

Bendich, Adrienne, Ph.D., and Charles Butterworth, M.D., eds. *Micronutrients in Health and Disease.* New York: Marcel Dekker, Inc., 1991.

> *Nutrition experts present the latest research findings on such issues as folic acid and the risk of cancer; vitamins B_6, B_{12} and folic acid and nerve or mental problems; and nutrients associated with age-related cataracts.*

Combs, Gerald F. Jr., Ph.D. *The Vitamins: Fundamental Aspects in Nutrition and Health.* San Diego: Academic Press, 1992.

> *Intended as a teaching text for an upper-level college course, this book offers background on the discovery of vitamins and details on their chemical structure.*

Composition of Foods. Washington, D.C.: Agricultural Research Services, U.S. Department of Agriculture, various dates.

> *The most recent series, number 8, includes 22 volumes that detail the nutrient content of thousands of foods: dairy and egg products, spices and herbs, baby foods, fats and oils, poultry products, soups, sauces and gravies, sausages and luncheon meats, breakfast cereals, fruits and fruit juices, pork products, vegetables and vegetable products, beef products and others.*

Diet and Health: Implications for Reducing Chronic Disease Risk. Food and Nutrition Board, Committee on Life Sciences, National Research Council. Washington, D.C.: National Academy Press, 1989.

> *This book, by the people who devise the RDAs, reviews current research linking various nutrients with chronic diseases, such as cancer and heart disease.*

Dommisse, J. "Subtle Vitamin B12 Deficiency and Psychiatry: A Largely Unnoticed but Devastating Relationship?" *Medical Hypotheses.* 34:2 (February 1991) 131-140.

The author uses reputably published literature—and extrapolations from it—to show that conditions like mood disorder, dementia, paranoid psychoses, violent behavior and fatigue are more commonly caused by B12 deficiency than currently is generally accepted.

Feltman, John, ed. *Prevention's Food and Nutrition.* Emmaus, Pa.: Rodale Press, Inc., 1993.

At 500-plus pages, this book offers easy reading on a wide variety of nutrition topics, including vitamins and minerals, fiber and fat.

Goodman, Kenneth I., M.D., and William B. Salt II, M.D. "Vitamin B12 Deficiency: Important New Concepts in Recognition." *Postgraduate Medicine.* 88:3 (September 1, 1990) 147-158.

A concise and complete review of the many possible causes and symptoms of B12 deficiency, and ways to accurately test for it.

Hausman, Patricia, R.D. *The Right Dose.* Emmaus, Pa.: Rodale Press, Inc., 1987.

Includes details on dosage levels at which vitamin and mineral supplements have been found to cause side effects, drug-nutrient and nutrient-nutrient interactions, nutrient interference with medical tests, and brand-by-brand comparisons of the common supplements found on drugstore shelves.

Heimburger, Douglas C., M.D., et al. "Improvement in Bronchial Squamous Metaplasia in Smokers Treated With Folate and Vitamin B12." *Journal of the American Medical Association.* 259:10 (March 11, 1988): 1525-1530.

A report of a study by researchers at the University of Alabama that found that folic acid and vitamin B12 reversed potentially premalignant lung cell changes in smokers.

Hendler, Sheldon Saul, M.D. *The Doctor's Vitamin and Mineral Encyclopedia.* New York: Simon and Schuster, 1990.

Along with providing good, practical advice, this carefully objective, readable book examines the claims made for just about every vitamin, mineral, herb and amino acid and other nutritional supplement on the market.

Miller, Benjamin, M.D., and Claire Brackman Keane, R.N. *Encyclopedia and Dictionary of Medicine, Nursing and Allied Health.* 5th ed. Philadelphia: W.B. Saunders, 1992.

A comprehensive, easy-to-understand dictionary of medical terms.

Morrill, Judi A., Ph.D. *Science, Physiology and Nutrition: A Primer for the Non-Scientist.* San Jose, Calif.: San Jose University Press, 1993.
> *Provides the basic science and physiology needed to understand certain aspects of nutrition, including easy-to-follow explanations of molecules, metabolism, digestion and the development of heart disease and cancer.*

Recommended Dietary Allowances. 10th ed. Food and Nutrition Board, Committee on Life Sciences, National Research Council. Washington, D.C.: National Academy Press, 1989.
> *From the people who figure the RDAs, a dry and sparse review of the function of each nutrient, food sources and usual dietary intake, and effects of deficiencies and excessive intakes. Includes tables for RDAs and suggested ranges.*

Reynolds, E.H., et al. "Multiple Sclerosis Associated With Vitamin B_{12} Deficiency." *Archives of Neurology.* 48:8 (August 1991) 808-811.
> *An intriguing look at the possible link between vitamin B_{12} deficiency and this serious nerve disorder, using actual case studies.*

Sauberlich, Howerde, and Lawrence J. Machlin, eds. *Beyond Deficiency: New Views on the Function and Health Effects of Vitamins.* Annals of the New York Academy of Sciences, Sept. 30, 1992. New York.
> *Research papers from leading experts in all areas of nutrition. Includes articles on the influence of AIDS on vitamin status and requirements, the relationship of vitamin C to blood pressure and cholesterol, and psychological disorders as early symptoms of vitamin deficiency, among many others.*

Stabler, Sally P., M.D., et al. "High Prevalence of Cobalamin Deficiency in Elderly Outpatients." *Journal of the American Geriatric Society.* 40:12 (December 1992) 1197-1204.
> *A study that confirms what many nutrition-oriented doctors have believed for years—that the incidence of B_{12} deficiencies in older people is significantly high.*

Stampfer, Meir J., M.D., et al. "Vitamin E Consumption and the Risk of Coronary Disease in Women." *New England Journal of Medicine* (May 20, 1993); 1444-1449.

Stampfer, Meir J., M.D., et al. "Vitamin E Consumption and the Risk of Coronary Disease in Men." *New England Journal of Medicine* (May 20, 1993); 1450-1456.
> *The original research findings that made the front page of the New York Times regarding vitamin E's apparent ability to slash the risk of heart disease in men and women.*

Weil, Andrew, M.D. *Natural Health, Natural Medicine.* Boston: Houghton Mifflin, 1990.
  A sensible guide to alternative medicine, including dietary recommendations and supplement use for numerous medical conditions.

Werbach, Melvyn. *Nutritional Influences on Illness.* 2nd ed. Tarzana, Calif.: Third Line Press, 1993.
  Abstracts and references of hundreds of studies relating to nutrition and illnesses, arranged by illness.

Werbach, Melvyn. *Nutritional Influences on Mental Illness.* Tarzana, Calif.: Third Line Press, 1991.
  Abstracts and references of hundreds of studies relating to nutrition and mental problems, such as aggressive behavior, alcoholism, anorexia nervosa, anxiety, autism, bipolar personality, insomnia, learning disorders, premenstrual syndrome and schizophrenia.

Many journals and newsletters are devoted to topics in nutrition. Among them:

American Journal of Clinical Nutrition
  Published by the American Society for Clinical Nutrition, it's the most prestigious of the nutrition-related professional journals. Includes first-time publication of research findings from around the world.

Journal of the American College of Nutrition
  Published by the American College of Nutrition, articles are mostly findings of research projects. Recent articles include the effect of zinc supplementation on people with eating disorders, risk factors for cardiovascular disease in children, and the effects of large doses of vitamin B6 on carpal-tunnel syndrome.

Journal of the American Dietetic Association
  The official publication of the American Dietetic Association, geared mostly toward dietitians. Current issues include articles on hospital-associated malnutrition, foods causing adverse reactions, and nutrition practices of people with AIDS.

The Journal of Optimal Nutrition
  A new periodical dedicated to publishing research findings and opinion regarding the optimal levels of nutrients in the diet and the body.

Nutrition Action Health Letter
  Easy-to-read short articles, food product reviews, and healthy recipes from the Center for Science in the Public Interest, in Washington, D.C.

Tufts University Diet and Nutrition Letter
  A reader-friendly review of current nutrition research. Recent issues include articles on why men gain weight after marriage, the hazards of raw milk, and why overweight people often underestimate the number of calories they consume.

APPENDIX A: Food and Nutrition Board, National Academy of Sciences—National Research Council Recommended Dietary Allowances,[a] Revised 1989

Designed for the maintenance of good nutrition of practically all healthy people in the United States

Category	Age (years) or Condition	Weight[b] (lb)	Height[b] (in)	Protein (g)	Fat-Soluble Vitamins				Water-Soluble Vitamins						
					Vitamin A (µg RE)[c]	Vitamin D (µg)[d]	Vitamin E (mg α-TE)[e]	Vitamin K (µg)	Vitamin C (mg)	Thiamin (mg)	Riboflavin (mg)	Niacin (mg NE)[f]	Vitamin B_6 (mg)	Folate (µg)	Vitamin B_{12} (µg)
Infants	0.0–0.5	13	24	13	375	7.5	3	5	30	0.3	0.4	5	0.3	25	0.3
	0.5–1.0	20	28	14	375	10	4	10	35	0.4	0.5	6	0.6	35	0.5
Children	1–3	29	35	16	400	10	6	15	40	0.7	0.8	9	1.0	50	0.7
	4–6	44	44	24	500	10	7	20	45	0.9	1.1	12	1.1	75	1.0
	7–10	62	52	28	700	10	7	30	45	1.0	1.2	13	1.4	100	1.4
Males	11–14	99	62	45	1,000	10	10	45	50	1.3	1.5	17	1.7	150	2.0
	15–18	145	69	59	1,000	10	10	65	60	1.5	1.8	20	2.0	200	2.0
	19–24	160	70	58	1,000	10	10	70	60	1.5	1.7	19	2.0	200	2.0
	25–50	174	70	63	1,000	5	10	80	60	1.5	1.7	19	2.0	200	2.0
	51+	170	68	63	1,000	5	10	80	60	1.2	1.4	15	2.0	200	2.0
Females	11–14	101	62	46	800	10	8	45	50	1.1	1.3	15	1.4	150	2.0
	15–18	120	64	44	800	10	8	55	60	1.1	1.3	15	1.5	180	2.0
	19–24	128	65	46	800	10	8	60	60	1.1	1.3	15	1.6	180	2.0
	25–50	138	64	50	800	5	8	65	60	1.1	1.3	15	1.6	180	2.0
	51+	143	63	50	800	5	8	65	60	1.0	1.2	13	1.6	180	2.0
Pregnant				60	800	10	10	65	70	1.5	1.6	17	2.2	400	2.2
Lactating	1st 6 months			65	1,300	10	12	65	95	1.6	1.8	20	2.1	280	2.6
	2nd 6 months			62	1,200	10	11	65	90	1.6	1.7	20	2.1	260	2.6

Category	Age (years) or Condition	Weight[b] (lb)	Height[b] (in)	Minerals Calcium (mg)	Phosphorus (mg)	Magnesium (mg)	Iron (mg)	Zinc (mg)	Iodine (µg)	Selenium (µg)
Infants	0.0–0.5	13	24	400	300	40	6	5	40	10
	0.5–1.0	20	28	600	500	60	10	5	50	15
Children	1–3	29	35	800	800	80	10	10	70	20
	4–6	44	44	800	800	120	10	10	90	20
	7–10	62	52	800	800	170	10	10	120	30
Males	11–14	99	62	1,200	1,200	270	12	15	150	40
	15–18	145	69	1,200	1,200	400	12	15	150	50
	19–24	160	70	1,200	1,200	350	10	15	150	70
	25–50	174	70	800	800	350	10	15	150	70
	51+	170	68	800	800	350	10	15	150	70
Females	11–14	101	62	1,200	1,200	280	15	12	150	45
	15–18	120	64	1,200	1,200	300	15	12	150	50
	19–24	128	65	1,200	1,200	280	15	12	150	55
	25–50	138	64	800	800	280	15	12	150	55
	51+	143	63	800	800	280	10	12	150	55
Pregnant				1,200	1,200	320	30	15	175	65
Lactating	1st 6 months			1,200	1,200	355	15	19	200	75
	2nd 6 months			1,200	1,200	340	15	16	200	75

Reprinted from RECOMMENDED DIETARY ALLOWANCES: 10TH EDITION. *Copyright 1989 by the National Academy of Sciences. Courtesy of the National Academy Press, Washington, D.C.*

[a] The allowances, expressed as average daily intakes over time, are intended to provide for individual variations among most normal persons as they live in the United States under usual environmental stresses. Diets should be based on a variety of common foods in order to provide other nutrients for which human requirements have been less well defined.

[b] Weights and heights of Reference Adults are actual medians for the U.S. population of the designated age, as reported by NHANES II. The median weights and heights of those under 19 years of age were taken from Hamill et al. (1979) (see pages 16–17). The use of these figures does not imply that the height-to-weight ratios are ideal.

[c] Retinol equivalents. 1 retinol equivalent = 1 µg retinol or 6 µg β-carotene. See text for calculation of vitamin A activity of diets as retinol equivalents.

[d] As cholecalciferol. 10 µg cholecalciferol = 400 IU of vitamin D.

[e] α-Tocopherol equivalents. 1 mg d-α tocopherol = 1 µTE. See text for variation in allowances and calculation of vitamin E activity of the diet as µ-tocopherol equivalents.

[f] 1 NE (niacin equivalent) is equal to 1 mg of niacin or 60 mg of dietary tryptophan.

APPENDIX B: SUMMARY TABLE
Estimated Safe and Adequate Daily Dietary Intakes of Selected Vitamins and Minerals[a]

Category	Age (years)	Vitamins		Trace Elements[b]					
		Biotin (μg)	Pantothenic Acid (mg)	Copper (mg)	Manganese (mg)	Fluoride (mg)	Chromium (μg)	Molybdenum (μg)
Infants	0–0.5	10	2	0.4–0.6	0.3–0.6	0.1–0.5	10–40	15–30
	0.5–1	15	3	0.6–0.7	0.6–1.0	0.2–1.0	20–60	20–40
Children and adolescents	1–3	20	3	0.7–1.0	1.0–1.5	0.5–1.5	20–80	25–50
	4–6	25	3–4	1.0–1.5	1.5–2.0	1.0–2.5	30–120	30–75
	7–10	30	4–5	1.0–2.0	2.0–3.0	1.5–2.5	50–200	50–150
	11 +	30–100	4–7	1.5–2.5	2.0–5.0	1.5–2.5	50–200	75–250
Adults		30–100	4–7	1.5–3.0	2.0–5.0	1.5–4.0	50–200	75–250

[a] Because there is less information on which to base allowances, these figures are not given in the main table of RDA and are provided here in the form of ranges of recommended intakes.

[b] Since the toxic levels for many trace elements may be only several times usual intakes, the upper levels for the trace elements given in this table should not be habitually exceeded.

Reprinted from RECOMMENDED DIETARY ALLOWANCES: 10TH EDITION. Copyright 1989 by the National Academy of Sciences. Courtesy of the National Academy Press, Washington, D.C.

INDEX